Two Trains Leave The Station

Two Trains Leave The Station

A Meditation on Aging, Alzheimer's, and Arithmetic

Catherine Landis

CLH

Cover design by Bruce Henschen, Sr.

Also by Catherine Landis

SOME DAYS THERE'S PIE

HARVEST

For My Father

Charles Francis Landis, Jr.

Education is more than learning a series of facts and tricks. It's building a citizen capable of critical thinking and confident of his or her abilities to solve problems.

Mary Smith

1

What if I'm stupid? How else to explain a 60-year-old woman who can't do math? It's hard not to feel stupid, walking around all these people who act like math is easy. So many people! Sixth graders! It's hard not to wonder. I don't like to talk about it because, you know, I don't want to sound stupid. Plus, it's easy to fake. Have I not managed to live a perfectly reasonable life without math? By math, of course, I mean ...

See? It's embarrassing. It's hard to say what I mean. I do not want to say it.

By math, I don't mean calculus. I don't even mean algebra. I mean: here's what I mean. When I started writing this book, friends wanted to know what I was up to.

What are you working on? What's it about?

Math, I told them. It's a book about math.

Math?

So then I would have to explain how I set out to learn as much math as possible and then write about the experience, a kind of math memoir, maybe, like a math meditation, but that only let to more questions.

What do you mean by math?

I mean, I don't remember how to multiply fractions.

That's arithmetic.

Right. I mean arithmetic.

Fractions, decimals, percentages. I seemed to remember there were tricks. Weren't there tricks? I had lost the tricks. And to be perfectly honest, the math facts. I'd lost some of those, too. Not all, but a few.

Quick: 5 x 4.

20!

The answer, instantaneous, like when you see blue, you know blue, but wait:

6 x 9?

That one didn't come so fast. I could get there but not instantly. I had to think for a bit, let the memory work through some muck that had gotten in the way.

There's a word for this, and it's not stupid. It's innumerate. Like illiterate but with math, and just how humiliating is that? I believe I would rather have all my clothes fall off in the middle of a crowded street than admit that third graders are better at math than I am, because if your clothes fall off, you can always put on more clothes, but when you can't do math? Something might be wrong with your brain. And if something is wrong with your brain, then something is wrong with you.

And yet third graders do math every day, do they not? As they did when they were first and second graders, as they will do for the next nine years, at least. They practice. When is it ever necessary for me use math? Never. Never is when I use math. Never is the number of times I have practiced math in more than 40 years.

But then never is also when I use a whole lot of what I learned in school. I cannot tell you the year the French Revolution started. I cannot name all the Presidents of the United States. I cannot locate Bulgaria on a map. I cannot remember the plot of *The Merchant of Venice*. Or *The Grapes of Wrath*. Or the titles of all the Yeats poems I used to love. Summarize the philosophy of Descartes? I'm not entirely sure I can. Name the parts of a cell? Not that either. What is entropy, where is iron on the periodic table, how long ago was the Cambrian Period? I used to know.

And every single bit of that I could know again with a few taps on my phone, and the fact that I would have to look it up would not be at all embarrassing to me. History, science, literature, philosophy, geography: all those subjects beg to be refreshed from time to time, but math is somehow not like that. Math feels like something I should just know. Elementary, like reading. Basic. Fundamental. Embodied knowledge. You don't have to remember how to read, why should it be different with math?

Because!!! I read every single day. The last time I multiplied two fractions together, I was 16 years old. Does this mean I should maybe give myself a break?

It's still embarrassing.

The year I turned 60, I was not happy or well behaved. My birthday is in June, and that winter and spring I devolved into an indignant, whining, stubborn, seething specimen of denial. If somebody had handed me a tool to stop time, I believe I would have used it.

Forty was not nearly this bad. Forty was even a sort of relief. Turning 40 felt like becoming fully adult, finally leaving behind some of the idiocy of my youth. At 40 you can pass for 35, you can still be young but wiser. Then came 50.

Turning 50 was like being pushed through a door I did not want to go through. There's no pretense of young in 50 unless it's "young-at-heart," which carries a whiff of platitude meant to bolster the spirits of the runners-up. I was forced to reconcile with the signs of aging cells: what's this loose chicken-skin above my knees and elbows, and where the hell did this belly come from, and are those jowls? But the real problem with 50 was the math. I had crossed a line where more than half of my life was over. Statistically speaking, of course. Who knows, I may have passed it at 40, I'm just talking odds here. It's something you can say with confidence at 50 that you don't at 30. You just don't. What then is there to say about that line at 60?

Goddammit.

Of course, I got used to 50, as one does. Fifty could even be fun when people would look at me and exclaim, *you don't look that old!* Ha, ha! Great fun. I'm not hearing that one so much anymore. As my 60th birthday approached, and I was operating just one level below full-on tantrum, I wasn't getting a lot of sympathy. A great many of my friends are older than I am, and I was complaining? My friend Mary, who would turn 70 later that same year, said it was a waste of time to think about age. My friend Grier, who would be turning 70 three days before I turned 60, was genuinely surprised. Didn't I know: the older you get, the better! You're freer, she told me. More yourself. Calmer and possibly kinder, less willing to put up with bullshit, but also more appreciative.

She was right, of course she was. I told her so, I said, "You're right!" But I was still working the math. "I just can't help feeling time is running out," I said, struggling to explain.

"Just be thankful for every day you're alive," she said.

I told her I would try.

But I didn't try. Instead, I doubled down on stubborn and decided to train for a half-marathon.

It's important to know that this half-marathon business was in direct opposition to the decision I had made years earlier never to do such a thing. At 25, I'd run a full marathon, and it was hard, and there was no reason to do it ever again. Not even half of it. At 59, I was regularly running a safe and comfortable five miles, two to three times a week, and that was enough. Plenty. It was sustainable for my goal to be running a comfortable five miles, two to three times a week, for the rest of my life. A healthy goal. Admirable. Achievable. How foolish to risk injury by pushing for more! Unnecessary. Imprudent. Ridiculous! I decided to do it anyway. Running a half-marathon would be my personal "fuck-you" to 60.

Want to keep from turning 60? Die first. It's really the only way.

My whine-fest stopped one evening in a restaurant in Sacramento, California, where we'd gone with my son Charlie, and his wife Alex, and Alex's mother, Tracey, a smart, strong, vibrant, and beloved woman in the fourth year of a fight against stage-4 breast cancer. Tracey would turn 55 later that summer. At dinner that night, I found myself regaling the table with my fuck-you-to-60 plan to run a half-marathon story, but when everybody laughed, I suddenly didn't. I was wishing I'd kept my mouth shut. Sitting next to Tracey, who could not say for certain that she would make it to 60, I understood how very not funny I was.

And so I stopped complaining. Just like that.

The year I turned 60 turned out to be a particularly momentous year but only partly because of my milestone birthday. It was the year when I did, indeed, run that first half-marathon and then another. It was the year I became a grandmother. And it was the year my smart, funny, beautiful mother was diagnosed with Alzheimer's disease.

And that was what finally did it. If my mother had Alzheimer's, I would have to discard pride, admit that I was, if not stupid, then innumerate, and make up my mind. It was time to learn some math.

1 + 1

Why math?

Innumeracy has never once kept me from doing a single thing. Innumeracy is not even remotely like illiteracy. Can't read? That's hard, really hard, like every day would be a struggle, but life without math? It's kind of shocking how little you actually need to know to get along in the world. And evidently, I'm not alone. To write this book, I ended up talking to dozens of people about math and found a staggering number of otherwise intelligent people who hate it, can't do it, never could do it, and shudder at the mere sound of the word, *fractions*. I don't know whether to be worried or happy for the company.

Statistics are tricky because it depends on who gets measured, who's doing the measuring, and when the measuring takes place, but it appears that more people are bad at math than good, at least in this country. Some researchers bemoaning this fact aim to prove there's a better way to teach this stuff, and there are a bunch of theories, philosophies, and strategies claiming to know just how to do that. Others warn of larger societal harms that come from innumeracy, like when people confuse correlation with causality, or see meaningless patterns in random events, or fear a shark attack more than the much likelier car accident, or don't understand exponential growth, as in, for instance, a global pandemic. Researchers look at innumeracy as a problem to solve.

I can't speak for anybody else, but the fact that I couldn't add two fractions together bugged the crap out of me. Whenever I found myself standing in front of a rack of shirts trying to figure out the final price on a 40 percent off sale, I'd get hit with a fresh wave of shame. Shame well earned, as it turns out. *How do you even live*, said one friend when she heard just how innumerate I was.

But you can carry around a little bit of shame for an awfully long time without doing anything about it. Shame was not a strong enough motivator for me to change. My mother's Alzheimer's was. That was the tipping point. That was the spark that turned shame into urgency.

Can learning something new keep you from losing your mind?

What about learning math?

Some studies have suggested that making your brain learn new things, especially hard things, may delay the onset of Alzheimer's for those at risk of getting the disease. Or it may not. But since it can't hurt, why not try? That's what I was thinking. You see a train speeding toward you, you may not want to just stand there. You may want to think about moving off the track.

My mother had been showing signs of forgetfulness for about two years before the official diagnosis. I'm guessing about two years because it's hard to pin down exactly when it started. Forgetfulness is not a disease, otherwise I've got it, and most likely you do, too. With the clarity of hindsight now, I remember one particular day when my mother called to tell me her dog was sick. There was nothing unusual about that, only the next day she called to tell me again, using exactly the same words to say exactly the same thing. It was almost as if she did not remember that she'd called the day before. At the time, it sounded only slightly weird. My mother was repeating herself more than usual, but that seemed to fall within a range of normal until gradually something else began to seem askew, an extra something I could not put my finger on. One particular summer morning during a visit with my folks, my father and I were up early talking in the kitchen, and for some reason it seemed like a good time to say out loud what I'd been thinking.

Is Mother getting more forgetful?

My dad's face crumpled; I'll never forget it. As crumples go, his was quick and slight but enough to let me know he'd been worrying in silence for who knows how long. He sounded somewhat relieved to finally speak the words he had been resisting. Just that morning, he told me, he'd discovered she'd left the garden hose on all night long.

It is not like my mother to leave the hose on all night. This is a woman who never leaves a door unlocked, much less open. She closes kitchen cabinets, returns books to bookshelves, hangs clothes back in the closet, folds shirts, and does not leave shoes in the middle of the floor all over the house. If anyone in the family can be considered careless and absent-minded, it's me. Not my mother.

She walked into the kitchen as my dad and I were talking. *What are y'all talking about?*

Your memory, said my dad, in a way that indicated they might have discussed this issue before.

She shrugged. "What are you going to do about it?" she said.

So. That's one way to look at it. Certainly not the way I would have expected. Wasn't she worried? Afraid? Sad? If she was, she was not letting on.

Later that day, my Dad and I resumed our conversation about my mother's increasing forgetfulness and this "something extra" I was sensing. What was it? I was searching for a word when my father nailed it. She's acting *old*, he said.

Old. It was not like my mother to act *old*.

I did not want this to be happening to my beautiful mother. How could this be the plan for the last years of her life? It was a terrible plan. Alzheimer's was the exact opposite of what was supposed to happen to her. I mean, it did happen, all the time, to other people, but not to my mother. We had not yet taken that trip to New York we'd so often talked about, and what about that cruise to Antarctica my dad was hoping for, and there was so much more jazz technique she was planning to learn on the piano, and there would be a new great grandson to play with. My mother was not the sort of person to grow old. She was very nearly famous for looking and acting younger than her age. Everybody said so. At 80, she looked 70 and acted 40: why should 90 be any different?

A moment that sticks out as I type these words recalls a summer afternoon in the living room of my parents' house where I was talking to an old friend who'd come over for a visit. Her mother had recently died. My mother was out, perhaps to a lunch date or a meeting of the board of directors of AVA, the arts organization she helped found. When she returned she walked into the living room to say hello to my friend, and the effect of her walking into that room, or any room, induced an involuntary gasp. She was thin and beautiful, wearing an aqua dress, always a great color on her, with a skirt made up of tiny pleats that fell just above her knees and shimmied around her still gorgeous legs. She would have had on expensive pumps with a slight heel and a touch of jewelry. She was animated. Thrilled to see my friend. Energized by wherever she'd been. Full of sharp humor and interesting observations. She was a sparkler that lit up the room, unquenchable. She was 80.

Now at 83, bam, she was old.

It felt that sudden. It would be another year before we'd find out why.

The official diagnosis, straight from the mouth of a neurologist, came the following June, four days before my 60thbirthday. Hearing the word, Alzheimer's, was upsetting and unsettling but it was also oddly comforting, a bitter relief to finally get an answer to what the hell was going on with Mother. When the doctor called with the news, my mother made a joke. "And who are you?" she asked when he'd finished explaining the test results. He started to repeat himself, "This is doctor ..." before realizing what she was doing. "That's a good one," he said. She laughed. We all laughed, but it wasn't really funny.

You hear Alzheimer's, and there are a couple of things you know. Mother is not going to get better, that's the first thing. How bad it might get, nobody knows. I knew it would be hard. Hard on her but mostly hard on my dad. Hard on my brother. Hard on me.

Here's another thing I knew: I might have to do something about my own brain.

The brain is a scary body part. You can't see it working. Or feel it. You can't know if or when some little thing might be going awry. I suppose that's the case for most of our internal organs but somehow the brain feels more precarious, more fragile, more personal. It's the *you* inside of you. The me inside of me. And like a first-year medical student hypochondronizing every internal twinge and twitch, I began imagining sensations inside my head: fogginess, stickiness, heaviness, slowness. Were these signs? Should I be worried? If my brain contained the genetic key that had turned on in my mother's brain, I wanted to stop it. It was time to put my brain on an exercise routine.

Of course, brain exercises are kind of a big deal these days. Like you can read about them in the *New York Times*. Like ads for them pop up above email inboxes. And every other day offers up a new study, a new program, a new magic elixir. Eat this, don't eat that, run, lift, stretch, sleep, don't stress out, and buy the newest brain game. There are several you can pay real money for to download onto your phone. They've become part of the scolding culture, the dire warnings that you better get your ass in gear or else. If you're doing what you're supposed to do, if you're living right, if you're a good girl and not a worthless scumbag, then you're eating your vegetables, juicing god knows what-all, cutting out sugar, sleeping 8 hours a night, and making sure that brain of yours never gets lazy. Make it work!

Digging down below the hype, the headlines, and the marketing, you find out that brain exercise doesn't necessarily mean a fancy game. It means making your brain do something it isn't used to. Crossword puzzles are popular, and they can work, but only if you're not used to working crossword puzzles. The trick is to learn something new: a musical instrument, a foreign language, an unfamiliar skill. Math? These are the tools for building more resilient brains. Maybe. The science is murky.

So far as I have been able to ascertain, no studies have shown evidence that anything can prevent Alzheimer's. None. Although a few suggest ways to slow the onset and progression. Actual physical exercise seems to be the most promising, but mental exercises offering novelty and complexity also might or might not help. In a group of people identified as Superagers -- older than 70 but with a

25-year-old's memory and attention – working *hard* appears to be a key. This I read in a December 2016 *New York Times* column: *How to Become a Superager*, by Lisa Feldman Barrett, professor of psychology at Northeastern University. In one study, Dr. Barrett teased out differences between Superagers and everybody else, which included, "Vigorous exercise and bouts of strenuous mental effort." As an example of strenuous mental effort, she suggested solving math problems.

Math. She probably wasn't talking about multiplying fractions. But might it be true that one person's arithmetic is another person's calculus?

Dr. Lee Lindquist, a Gerontologist at Northwestern University's Feinberg School of Medicine, has done research with older patients indicating that exercise and "active learning" may at least slow down cognitive decline in Alzheimer's and other dementias. "We're all worried we're going to be the next to get Alzheimer's," Dr. Lindquist told me. "And we're all asking: *What can I do to beat this?*"

No shit.

It's a generational thing, she added. "Baby boomers never really embraced growing old. Baby boomers as a group have always tried to kind of rebel against everything, and I think aging is one more way of rebelling. I see among the 80 and 90-year-olds the attitude of: *this is my life. Put me in a nursing home when I need to go.* But I see the 60 and 70-years-olds being like: *I'm going to beat this. I'm not going to age. I'm not going to get memory loss. I'm going to do everything I can to avoid it.*"

Exactly.

Why math? That's why.

One hot July day I found myself in a parking lot in front of a School Box store two doors down from the shoe store where I'd gone looking for shoes. I didn't find the shoes, but walking back to my car, I caught myself staring at the bright yellow School Box sign. What is a School Box store? I had no idea, but presumed it sold school supplies, and as I stood in the parking lot staring at the sign, I could not help wondering how long was I going to keep talking about what I maybe ought to do one of these days.

I don't know what I was expecting, something brightly lit and cheery like its sunny yellow sign on the outside, but the School Box was low-ceilinged and dimly lit with a flea market, general store feel. There was a whiff of Christian indoctrination. Was this where home-schooling parents shopped for academic materials? INSPIRATION was one of the sections marked by homemade signs hanging from the ceiling. I looked for the sign for MATH.

A basic workbook might be a way to start, but which grade? I had no idea. Two matching Kelly green third grade workbooks caught my eye, one for multiplication, one for division. It was as good a start as any. Walking toward the checkout counter, I decided to pretend to be buying these books for a kid, if anybody asked. Nobody asked. I paid for the workbooks, scurried back to the car, and snuck them into the house. This was real. This was happening. The ticket bought, the bags packed, I was on my way. Sixty-year-old woman, learning math.

That afternoon I took the workbooks outside to the screen porch to begin what I was calling my grand math project in the reassuring company of cicadas and warring hummingbirds, but I did not open them. Instead I took a pencil and a blank piece of paper and wrote out my own multiplication table, working off a theory that the physical act of moving a pencil by hand to mark a number on a page might open a line to memory, similar to how the physical act of writing sentences generates ideas more efficiently for me than sitting around, thinking. Who knows if the theory holds up, but my multiplication exercise was revealing.

I wrote my math facts in vertical rows, even the ones I knew: the ones, the twos, the threes, the fours, up to the tens, and most of them I *saw*. 5 x 3. *15*. I *saw* it instantly. But 4 x 7? I didn't *see* 28, not right away, and 7 x 8, I didn't *see* anything at all. There were holes in the fabric of my memory. Six of them. Here were my holes:

4 x 7

6 x 8

6 x 9

7 x 8

7 x 9

8 x 9

Clearly, if I had any hope of successfully relearning math I was going to have to fix this. I made flash cards but then remembered I'm the sort of person who appears to learn better when somebody explains things to me. Might that suggest I'm an audio learner? So before attempting the flash cards, I recorded myself singing the times tables into my phone. All I'd have to do is play it back and those pesky facts would stick in my brain!

Only it didn't work. Listening to math facts is boring. I tuned them out, daydreamed, made grocery lists. Swimming laps in my neighborhood pool the next morning, I ran through the math facts in my head: 25 meters of multiplying 6's, 25 meters for 7's, and so on, and as I swam and multiplied I reconsidered. It could be that I am, in fact, an audio-learner when it comes to microwave instructions and driving directions, but a visual learner when it comes to numbers. To me, numbers come in colors. 1: pale yellow, 2: blue, 3: green, 4: bright yellow, 5: red, 6: French blue, 7: golden, 8: purple, 9: black, 10: white. And while numbers beyond 10 don't appear in specific colors, there is still a strong visual component to them in my head. Forty-two, consisting of a yellow 4 and a blue 2, makes me *see* a sunny day at the beach. Thirty-four is sunlight streaming through a summer forest. Fifty-six is the French flag.

Allow me to pause here to say that I understand how strange this might sound. I understand that not everybody sees numbers in color and that, of those who do, their colors don't necessarily line up with mine. I understand that listening to people at a dinner party arguing over whether 5 is red or green can be tedious and irritating. Still, I can know only what I know, and I've never once seen a number that wasn't in color, but until that morning I had not considered the idea that learning math might have a strong visual connection for me.

The math facts came back fast. I gave myself a week to memorize them; it ended up taking only about a half a day, but you know what really helped? Like, no kidding, really helped? Practice. I opened my workbooks and practiced, 15 minutes a day, over and over, and I did get better, but I also discovered something I had not expected. It was, in fact, the absolute last thing I would have predicted, given how much frustration and anxiety I'd felt as a child learning math. Working math problems is strangely relaxing. Calming. Meditative. I was flabbergasted.

Math is meditative. Evidently this radical concept is common knowledge to some people, including my daughter-in-law, Liz, who nodded vigorously when I mentioned it one night over dinner. Liz said she loved math when she was a kid, and not only that, she absolutely does remember it as being calming and centering. Like working a puzzle, she said.

Indeed. You would not believe how many people talk about puzzles when they talk about math. IT'S LIKE A PUZZLE, I was told, over and over, as if that explained everything, a self-evident fact that proves math is awesome, like ice cream. But can I say I've ever cared for puzzles? No, I cannot. I'd rather rake leaves than work a puzzle. Perhaps that's part of the problem.

And yet it's hard to deny that the calming and centering aspects Liz spoke of made sense in that math is one of those things that forces you to slow down, to live in the moment. She has fond memories of working math problems with her dad and so her relationship with math carries positive emotional resonance. She'll also concede that math came easy for her. As it did for my sons, as it did for their dad. And my dad, as well as my mother, come to think of it, and my brother and a great many of my friends. I'm not sure how it happened, but I find myself surrounded by mathematically inclined people. Way before they stepped foot in a school, my kids were thinking about numbers in ways, I swear, I never have. I remember an afternoon when Charlie was 3, he lined up four yellow blocks and six blue blocks and then informed me that 4 and 6 must – logically -- equal 10.

Was this normal? Not to me. His older brother Bruce was entertaining himself in the backseat of the car by working math problems in his head, and that didn't seem normal either. When they did get to school, they never asked for help. There are no memories in this family of sitting down with Dad or anybody else to work math problems. Math was the easy homework.

To my great astonishment, I discovered that more than a few of my friends have fond memories of learning math. Certainly not all of them. A handful report hating math even more than I did, but most swear they enjoyed it, and many considered it fun. Fun! Even more astonishing: friends who were not particularly good in math; they thought it was fun, too, like working puzzles.

Again with the puzzle thing! Who knew so many people loved puzzles.

Even my friend Christy who, like me, tended to be more comfortable and somewhat gifted in the English/literature world. Christy, also like me, went to Wilkes T. Thrasher Elementary School on Signal Mountain, Tennessee, where we learned our multiplication tables in third grade. Christy had Mrs. Tate for third grade, a teacher so intimidating that Christy remembers enduring the pain of appendicitis for hours until her mother picked her up after school because she was too afraid of Mrs. Tate to tell her she was hurting. I wasn't lucky enough to have Mrs. Tate. I had Mrs. Atwater. The mention of her name terrifies me still.

I can close my eyes and place myself in my assigned seat on the right half of the room about four rows back at my little desk with the cubbyhole underneath that was messy all the time. Not everybody's was messy. I'm guessing Betty Moss's desk was always neat and orderly. To me, that was a mystery. Not only did I not know how mine got so messy, I had no idea how to keep it from getting that way. There appeared to be some secret involving papers that remained flat, straight, and neatly stacked, while mine ended up wrinkled, rumpled, wadded up, and crammed into the innards of the cubbyhole where I could not find them without a panicked search. Mrs. Atwater disapproved of messy desks, and I vaguely remember getting in trouble for it. Not the worst kind of trouble: Mrs. Atwater hung a wooden paddle on the wall at the front of the classroom and she used it -- never on me, but the threat was always there. For me, trouble might have entailed staying in at recess to clean out my desk, but I was a good girl and could barely endure the humiliation of getting in trouble for anything. I also resented it. It felt like being punished for something I couldn't help.

Mrs. Atwater was an old woman. I don't know that this is true. For all I know, she was no more than 40, but when I was eight, my mother was 32, and so I presume that anyone older than my mother looked old to me. She was old and mean and unfair because she gave me C's on my report card for penmanship, which was also humiliating and infuriating because it seemed to me that penmanship was one of those things like a tidy desk or pretty hair that some people have and some people don't. I could try or not try, the result was the same: my clumsy hands were incapable of forming beautiful letters. Mrs. Atwater's scornful C's made me feel ashamed and ugly. Mrs. Atwater was the teacher who taught me multiplication and division.

Did it matter? I don't know. In fifth grade, they pulled me and Christy and a handful of other classmates out of class for a special Great Books program. They were handing me books to read. They were making time in the day for us to discuss those books. They wanted to know what I had to say. In other words, read, discuss, repeat -- ask me what I would rather do, even now. But how did they know? Something about me made somebody think I could manage the Great Books program, so maybe I'm simply built this way? Born to be good at English and bad at math? Maybe it mattered not one bit who the teachers were.

Still, it is impossible for me not to wonder whether there might be significance in the fact that I learned key concepts in arithmetic from a woman who scared the living daylights out of me.

Then came Mrs. Haskins. Eighth grade.

Like Mrs. Atwater, my eighth-grade math teacher Mrs. Haskins was another old woman who might have only looked old to me but, instead of fear, this time my overwhelming emotion was outrage. In Mrs. Haskins' class, math became infuriating. Which math was that, exactly? I could not have told you until one day, as I was making my way through math workbooks and online videos, I came across a problem that went something like this:

Allie rides to the park on her bike. It takes her 24 minutes, going 8 miles an hour, peddling uphill the whole way. Coming home by the same route, she goes 18 miles per hour. What is her average rate of speed over the entire trip?

I had no idea. Can a person figure out the answer to a problem like this using the basic tools of arithmetic? I tried, but couldn't do it. The Khan Academy online lesson program I happened to be working on lets you ask for hints and so finally I gave up. What's my hint? I was instructed that the formula for finding the average rate of speed is total distance divided by total time.

Seriously? There's a formula? You have to know the formula to work the problem? I must have missed the formula. What if you forget the formula? I found myself wanting to know if there might be a logical way to arrive at the formula, I mean, somebody had to come up with it in the first place. Right?

And just like that, I'm back in eighth grade. The average rate of speed on a bike, in a car, in a canoe, two trains that leave some damn station: I'm talking about word problems that depend on formulas that my eighth-grade self was just supposed to remember even though they made zero sense to me.

But, wait: I was a word person! Wasn't I? I wrote poetry! I consumed books like an unrepentant addict! And there was old Mrs. Haskins with her arbitrary formulas speaking a language I did not understand and, I mean to tell you, it became my mission on earth to straighten her out. I argued with her. I demanded to know the meaning behind these formulas. I refused to believe anything she told me.

Or.

Maybe I couldn't get past the being scared I might not have it in me to understand.

Or.

Maybe I couldn't get past the anger that I was just supposed to accept the stupid rules and move on. Like everybody else.

When I say eighth grade came back to me, I don't just mean the math. Looking back with older eyes, I suspect the problem wasn't

Mrs. Haskins and it wasn't math. Eighth grade, 1969, I was 13 and walked around enraged all the time.

Maybe outrage is part of being 13 for everybody, I don't know. For me, that early adolescent phase of figuring out who you are got wrapped up in what was happening in the world, and what was happening in the world meant Vietnam, Civil Rights, and then Martin Luther King, Jr. was killed. I was horrified and upset, my parents were horrified and upset, but my grandparents were not. To me that proved that racism was generational. By my calculations, we had only to wait for the older people to die out and that would be the end of racism.

But then, in Mrs. Schmidt's eighth grade English class somebody said something. I don't remember what, but it must have indicated that some of my classmates were not thrilled by the ongoing and inevitable march toward racial justice, and I was shocked. How was racism ever going to end if this shit kept going on? The class discussion grew heated as I righteously defended the civil rights movement. No one has ever accused me of remaining calm in an argument. I was right, they were wrong; the impasse would not break until they yielded. Then one of the girls asked me if I would *marry* a black person.

Yes, I said. I would.

The class erupted in disbelief. By no means was I the only civil rights champion in that room, but I'd gone further than the rest, which got me teased and gawked at for a week or so. I don't think I cared.

Eighth grade, 1969, I was 13 and decided to be a girl who did not wear make-up. For context, from 7th through 12thgrade I went to a private girls' preparatory school, literally, Girls Preparatory School. GPS was founded in 1906, and the uniforms had not changed much since: short-sleeved cotton shift in any solid color, collared with a black grosgrain ribbon bow, tiny white buttons, and tiny pleats down the front, pulled together at the waist by a thin brown leather belt with a small brass colored GPS belt buckle. The standard joke was a tired cliché but it was also sort of true: the uniform made us look like we were wearing potato sacks, but I didn't mind. It was comfortable and easy and meant never having to stand in front of a closet wondering what to wear. White bobby socks were required, but we had a choice of saddle oxfords or loafers, (only saddle oxfords for me since my mother insisted loafers were bad for my feet). Ostentatious jewelry and make-up were forbidden. Unofficially, we wore colorful petty pants, hiking our dresses up over the belt to show them off under the hem. Twice a year on "civilian day" we could wear anything we wanted.

Just one year later, changes in culture and fashion would make it down to provincial Chattanooga, and civilian day would mean wearing jeans and dressing down, but when I was in eighth grade it meant dressing up. Mini-skirts and plaid jumpers and ruffled blouses and fishnet stockings and heels and make-up. I had stashed the tools in a little purse -- lipstick, powder, rouge, mascara, blue eye shadow -- and between classes there was a rush to the bathroom to reapply. I suppose we were desperate to maintain our newly discovered grown-up faces. Either that or we were showing off how grown-up we were in front of each other. I remember desperation. I remember being worried that I didn't know how to do it right, this make-up routine, while the other girls seemed to be pros. I remember the crowded bathroom and me standing in the back of the crowd, five or six girls deep, jostling for a clear view of the mirror, jostling and yearning to be beautiful. A flick of the mascara brush to lengthen the lashes, a slash of pink on the lips, a touch up of powder on the nose. I was jostling. I was desperate.

Then suddenly, like an epiphany, really, I had one clear thought: boys don't have to do this. Boys, in fact, would not put up with this shit. Boys walk around barefaced and nobody suggests they aren't attractive. I put the lipstick back in my purse, resolved: anybody who doesn't like the way I look? Tough. This is me, take it or leave it. Don't like my face? Not my problem. Who wants to hang around superficially judgmental people anyway? I walked into that bathroom yearning to be beautiful and walked out an unapologetic feminist, and I did not wear make-up again until my wedding day in 1982 when my mother asked, "Can I please just put a little color on your lips?"

Sure.

Eighth grade, 1969, I was 13 and in the middle of my short-lived but intense religious phase in which I sensed there was SOMETHING OUT THERE BIGGER THAN ME and Jesus was my best friend. The Jesus of 1969 was all about love, and my Jesus was the radical warrior fighting racism, the Vietnam War, poverty, patriarchy, hypocrisy, and capitalism. I could be a warrior, too, if I dedicated my life to Jesus. I read the entire Bible on my own. I looked for signs. I prayed for help in resisting the temptation to gossip. I wrote poems aimed at pinning down my inexplicable spiritual feelings. I kept my religious fervor to myself for the same reason that you don't brag about money or anything else that might give you unfair advantage over others, but alone I spent hours after school sitting on a rock across the street from my house on the edge of Signal Mountain overlooking Chattanooga, talking to Jesus, writing poetry, longing to catch a glimpse of god in the trees, and wishing I could be a better person.

This was the righteous, feminist, Jesus-freak eighth grader who sat in Mrs. Haskin's math class, demanding to know what the heck she was talking about. Two trains leaving the station? What was the point? Where was the underlying purpose? What connection could some arbitrary *formula* have to any of this, and anyway, couldn't formulas be considered a kind of cheating? And why was no one else outraged? It's possible all of us were, every single girl in my class, every 13-year-old everywhere, if not outraged then at least stuck in a mire of confusion, but I appeared to be the only one taking it out on poor Mrs. Haskins.

Eventually my mother intervened. I don't remember what she said to Mrs. Haskins the day she went to school to talk to her -- my mother doesn't remember either -- but whatever it was, it must have worked. Something did, because Mrs. Haskins and I slowly began to understand each other and by the spring I had quit fighting her. I have a vague memory of a brief period of time when I began to see that math might not be so horrible. It might even be fun. (Not puzzle fun, just plain fun.)

So many of my friends talk about *that one teacher* who inspired them to love math, who changed the way they thought about math forever after that, and I have wondered if Mrs. Haskins could have been that teacher for me in another place and time. Who knows. Maybe if we'd had more time. I can't say Mrs. Haskins had any permanent effect on my relationship to math, but I will say that she briefly broke through the barriers of rage and insecurity and fear that I had built between math and me, and by the end of the year I was doing much better in math class. I believe I may have pulled out an A. I believe I even apologized to Mrs. Haskins. I believe she smiled.

Mrs. Atwater, third grade, and Mrs. Haskins, eighth grade: two points on an otherwise bland and forgettable line of math classes I endured. Where on that line would it have predicted that I would grow up to be innumerate? After Mrs. Haskins, I took Algebra I in 9th grade, geometry in 10th grade, and Algebra II in 11th grade, each dissolving into the same bland line. I remember almost nothing of math from those years. I don't even remember the names of my teachers. I do remember that for our senior year we were given a choice: calculus or advanced American History, and all my friends chose calculus. Not just Jane and Mary Katherine, who wound up becoming doctors, or Karen, who went on to major in math in college, but Christy, who majored in English and French, and Lindsay, who studied Latin and Greek. For Lindsay, calculus was an exercise in self-improvement.

Not for me. I was done. I never took another math class for the rest of my life.

$$2(6+4)/4$$

I am 60 years old, sitting at my kitchen table working math problems, when it occurs to me that numbers are not just numbers. They stand for something in the real world. They are symbols. At its core, the number 3 is not a green abstraction sitting in its place on a number chart. It's three apples. Three pencils. Three trees. Three fingers. Math is a language, that's all, just another language we can use to interpret the world and communicate certain ideas. Evidently many six-year-olds understand this, but I was not one of those six-year-olds. Even you might be reading this and thinking, *duh*. When I mentioned it to Bruce, the look on his face was as if I'd told him that I had just discovered fire is hot. Why was I just now figuring this out?

Did you know: 4(3+5) is the same thing as 12 + 20? Of course you did.

Or maybe you didn't.

I am aware that some readers may have justifiably thrown this book across a room, because who wants to read about some idiot who has to bone up on math facts? But I also suspect that some people reading this are thinking *thank god I'm not alone.* If you're one of those people, then you might know what I mean when I say *I sort of knew* 4(3+5) is the same thing as 12 + 20. But I didn't really. It's one of those things I could have guessed was probably true. And certainly I could have worked it out, adding 3+5 to get 8, multiplying that by 4 to get 32, the same as 12 + 20, so I would have gotten there eventually. I could have proved the why of how the damn thing works. But I did not own the underlying concept of why. It was not in my core. No doubt it was a simple concept I knew once, then lost, but was it lost because I never did understand it in a deep way, or is it merely an example of you lose what you don't use? For whatever reason, math never once meant anything to me but a series of tricks and formulas I was told to memorize in order to manipulate these abstract numbers. If you forget the tricks: you can't do the math.

Fractions were my wall. All those years when I secretly worried that I could not do math, I would specifically be referring to the fact that I did not remember how to work with fractions. Everything on this side of the wall, no problem, but on the other side stretched a vast territory inhabited by decimals, percentages, statistics, probability, algebra, geometry, and darkness. Subjects so out of reach I could not see them. But until I conquered fractions, there was no point in even trying to get there.

Fractions are a hurdle for lots of people, and teachers have told me it's the hardest thing to get kids to remember. I came across a November 2017 *Scientific American* article by Robert S. Siegler that confirmed my hunch: the problem is widespread, at least in this country, where studies show children in the United States do much worse on standard fraction problems than children in many other countries. One problem, Siegler writes, is how inherently crazy fractions are.

Indeed. I am compelled to pause for a moment to note how heartening it is to read in no less than *Scientific American* that maybe there is a little something *inherently crazy* going on with fractions.

For starters, of course, you have to get the same denominator when adding and subtracting but not when multiplying and dividing, and in division you have to do this flipping thing between the numerator and denominator, a trick that feels very close to cheating or magic, depending on your point of view. None of this is hard once you learn how to do it but, apparently and according to these studies, it's easy to forget it.

Yes, it is.

Language, Siegler goes on to say, is one culprit. Some languages express fractions such as 2/3 not as *two thirds* but *out of three, two.* Such a turn of words would stick in your head in a different way, would it not? Such a clever and valiant tool to snatch numbers out of the intangible cloud of abstraction. As a solution, Siegler recommends teaching teachers more sustainable ways to teach fractions.

Sounds good. A little late for me.

Here was my big surprise. It didn't take me long to break down the fraction wall. It was, in fact, anti-climactic. I'd set myself up for a brutal and sustained attack and then it took, I don't know, maybe 20 minutes to knock it down? I did not remember that I knew how to find a least common denominator and all the rest, but the knowledge was there, waiting for me to come find it again. How many things are lying dormant in the brain, things we used to know but don't anymore? For a moment I allowed myself to wonder if this math project was going to be easy.

The moment passed. Quickly it became clear the difference between knowing how and doing. Struggling to convert fractions to decimals, for instance. Or slogging through to the end of a word problem only to find out I'd multiplied the fractions wrong. Or later, making mistake after mistake in the arithmetic for an algebraic equation that otherwise I would have solved. You can know how fractions work but still have trouble working with them. In those first heady days I had no idea how much practice it was going to take for these old forgotten skills to become second nature.

But at least I had the basics.

Until I didn't. Sometimes, I swear, my brain just spazzes out.

I am working through an online lesson. I am looking at the problem: 2/5 x 5/9. Easy! I know, I know! We're talking multiplying and simplifying, that's it. I've done it dozens of times now without an instant of skepticism, but I'm watching the video and the instructor is demonstrating how to cancel out those 5's to get the answer – JUST CANCEL THEM OUT! -- and suddenly I'm not happy. My heart is racing. Why? I'm starting to get pissed off, and my mind is seizing a little bit. Is this a trick?

If it's a trick, then how does it work? Why does it work? I'm staring at this guy and feeling like he's trying to get me to take this stuff on faith, and I'm not good at taking anything on faith. I am not a faith-based thinker.

I pause the video to work the problem the long way: multiplying the 2 x 5 in the numerator and then the 5 x 9 in the denominator, and that gets me to 10/45, which simplifies to 2/9, which is exactly the same thing you'd get if you cancel those 5's.

So. Does that mean I proved the point? Does that mean I can accept that the canceling trick works and just do it?

I guess so. But it's alarming to think about how quickly I got in the way of myself. Maybe overthinking a little bit? Turning something easy into something hard?

So many blips on my way toward joining the tribe of people who are not afraid of fourth grade math. I will concede, I have mixed feelings about it. I'm happy to know I can manage fractions now, exceedingly happy and relieved and even a little proud, but I'm also finding myself protective of the little girl I used to be, given instructions on how to work with fractions, given worksheets to complete, problems to solve, homework, tests, but no context. The lessons were shoved in her face and she was told to just do them. I feel in my bones what she was thinking.

WHY, she wanted to know.

She never did get an answer.

3(26-24)

I am watching my mother work crossword puzzles. She's pretty good. It is true my mother has always been good at crossword puzzles as she has been good at grammar, particularly good at spelling, at which I am not so good. The manipulation of words to unearth and articulate ideas, that's what I'm best at, my sustenance, my weapon, my shield, but not so much the grammar and spelling part of it, and certainly not crossword puzzles. In the same way I *see* numbers in color, my mother *sees* words in her mind, for instance, when she hears the word *success*, she *sees* S U C C E S S scrolling across her mind. It could be that's what makes her such a good speller. I don't *see* words scrolling across my mind. I hear them, but in a Southern accent, which turns out to be the opposite of helpful.

My mother cannot remember what I just told her or what she said to me five minutes ago. She can't call up all the words she wants to use in a sentence. She relies often on clichés, the same clichés over and over like training wheels on a bicycle that save her from falling mid-sentence. Lifelines she reaches for through a void. When I end a phone conversation by saying, "Well, that's all I know," I can count on her calling up Keats: *And all ye need to know.* As if it's the first time – and not the hundredth time -- she's thought to say it. Yet she can crack open a clue in a crossword puzzle and come out with an answer more often than her disintegrating memory would suggest possible. Does she remember why she started working crossword puzzles in the first place?

I don't know. It is so very hard to tell what my mother is thinking or how she is feeling and if she's hiding feelings of sadness over what is happening to her. She does not act sad or frightened. Often she appears confused but it does not seem to distress her, this confusion. This is so not like my mother.

My mother didn't used to be merely comfortable talking about her feelings; she talked about them all the time. She called me on the telephone: sometimes excited but more often frustrated, angry, or depressed, and often we parsed those emotions for what might lie underneath: inadequacy, fear, the helplessness of feeling unheard. It was part of the rhythm of our lives, this quest for clarity, for meaning, for connection, for healing, a drilling down into the what-the-hellness of our lives. These days she does not appear connected to those feelings. The quest has ended. Something has changed in who my mother is. Sharp edges have become rounded. A well is drying up. Like a roaming cell phone searching for a signal, there's an occasional sense that she's trying to figure something out but doesn't remember what. There's a sense that she's lost but doesn't know it.

I catch myself all the time wanting to go back and locate the moment when things changed. My mother's decline has been remarkably gradual. There's no telling how many tiny shifts we missed, how many we are missing still. When was the last honest conversation I had with her, when she and I operated as equals, bantering, debating, conversing, woman to woman, without me accommodating for her diminishing self? I want so badly to remember. To mark, to memorialize, to hold to my heart a precious moment that I had no way of knowing was precious until it was gone.

I'm not sure she always remembers she has Alzheimer's. We do talk about it. From the beginning, my dad has not wavered from his intention to preserve her dignity and autonomy. If there are decisions to be made, she's in on them. She hates it when we talk about her behind her back, and so when we do, we're careful she doesn't find out. We talk openly about the Alzheimer's and frequently she'll crack the same joke –*now who are you?*

For a good while after she was diagnosed she had the presence of mind to object when my dad would tell their friends about it. I'm venturing to say that more of her ego was operating at that time. And my father was willing to go along with her for quite a while, until the memory loss became noticeable.

Why is Charlotte asking the same question five times in a row?

If you know she has Alzheimer's, you're going to smile and answer five times. If not, you're just going to be confused. Also annoyed. So it was kinder, really, to let their friends know what was up with Charlotte. I once tried to explain that to her, to help her understand why my father felt the need to tell the truth.

She nodded and said, yes, yes, she understood all about Alzheimer's, then added, "But I don't have it *yet!*"

When you are confused, do you feel it? Can you be lost but not know it? If your capacity for thinking narrows, how would you know? We *can* know only what we *do* know. My mother may or may not remember that she started working crossword puzzles to keep her mind sharp and her memory clear. I don't think it's working, but there's no point in telling her. There's nothing wrong with crossword puzzles.

49-42

On a morning in August, I am standing in Lucy Tyler's second grade classroom at the Episcopal School of Knoxville. Lucy is getting her room ready for the fall semester to start. I'm here to talk to her about how she teaches math, and I notice a nifty number grid on a poster hanging on the wall. Stacked vertically on the left are the numbers 1 – 12. The same numbers line up horizontally across the top. Just a glance at the poster, it is easy to see: if you want to multiply 6 times 7, for instance, you find the 6 on one line, the 7 on the other, then follow your fingers down and across until they meet at 42. It is stunningly logical.

Maybe you've seen such a chart before but I never had, at least as far as I can remember, and looking at it, I cannot not help wondering if kids learning math with such a grid on the classroom wall would end up with something like it as the number chart in their minds. I mention this as a possibility to Lucy. She doesn't know what I'm talking about.

"If my number chart looked like that grid, math might have been easier for me," I explain.

"What chart?"

I draw my number chart on the smart board.

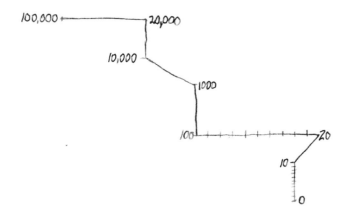

"I have no idea."

"Because it doesn't make any sense."

"I know! That's what I'm saying. What if one of the reasons math is hard for me is because my chart doesn't have any patterns. But on the grid, right there, you see patterns."

She continues to look at me as if suddenly I'd begun talking about elves. It is a significant pause. Several seconds. More than ten. She isn't saying anything. Finally I think to ask, "You don't have a number chart in your brain?"

"No," she says.

That evening I ask Bruce about his number chart. He doesn't know what I'm talking about.

It's hard to convey how stunned I was to hear this. Sixty years old and just learning that not everybody has a number chart. Not everybody sees numbers in color, either, and I knew that and had no trouble accepting it, but somehow the number chart is different. My chart is as stable and clear and foundational as the taste of salt, as the color blue, as the warmth of the sun on my skin. When I think 26, I *see* 26 in its place on my chart. It's so fundamental that I never bothered to ask anybody else where 26 might be located.

So I began asking. Family members and friends – any number charts? And guess what? Most people don't carry around number charts in their minds. My survey sample, per usual, was small and seriously unscientific, but in my little world there are more people without charts than with them. Again, I pause to emphasize the mind-blowing impact of this news. Imagine finding out that most of the people you know don't taste salt on their potato chips.

But could I be on to something? I was excited to maybe have stumbled on some reason for so wide a discrepancy in basic math ability. Could there be a correlation between number charts and sucking at math?

No. Some people who are quite skilled at math also have number charts in their brains, as it turns out. Number charts are not the same from person to person, and some number chart people see colors while others don't. Evidently all of this is a form of synesthesia, a perceptual phenomenon in which stimulation of one sensory pathway automatically stimulates a second sensory pathway. It can take a wide variety of forms, and I knew that and had always assumed that the minds of synesthetes were filled with explosive sounds and colors and smells, a cross-circuitry of senses gone crazy: hearing colors, smelling numbers, and other disturbing phenomena. All I've got is a handful of colorful charts in my brain, (numbers, decades, years, months in the year, days of the week), which suggests only one pathway stimulating another pathway, but somehow that makes me a synesthete.

Still the question: does it mean anything at all?

I will say this much. Teachers these days appear to be doing a better job than my teachers did at imparting basic concepts like— let's say -- place value. And it seems to me that if you get a real, gut-level, tangible, and unwavering understanding of place, then you know what 296 means. It means 200 plus 90 plus 6. That is very different from the way I see 296, a number with a blue-green tint perched on a horizontal line on its way from 100 up to 1,000. My chart is pretty. Mildly interesting. But nothing about it helps me understand what 296 means. So maybe? Yes? In some small way my number chart got between me and math. What else might have?

In her classroom that August morning, Lucy tells me there's not one way to teach math. "You use every kind of way you can think of," she says, "because what works for one student might not work for another." Like open response, the name she gives to the technique of encouraging students to come up with a variety of ways to solve a single problem To demonstrate, she goes to the smart board and writes:

26 + 48 = ?

She then shows me several different ways to solve it without having to know tricks like borrowing and carrying. Like you can add 25 and 50 to get 75, then add 1 and subtract 2. Or you can add 20 and 40, then 6 and 8, and then 60 and 14.

"I tell the kids it's like being a carpenter," Lucy says. "You want as many tools in your tool box as you can have because if you can't solve a problem using one, you have more to choose from."

So true, but all I can think is, I wish I'd had Ms. Tyler in second grade.

Alice remembers the nuns. They were her teachers in Catholic school who taught her, well, everything, but this is a book about math and so Alice and I were talking about math class. "It was boring," she told me, kind of laughing, but kind of not. "It was worksheets and a lot of pressure, and I was supposed to do it even if I didn't understand it. Teachers presented it only one way and that's how you did it. You just had to memorize. And then you had word problems, and everybody dreaded word problems. That's why I don't call them word problems in my class, I call them number stories, because who wants to do a *problem*?"

Indeed. Alice Ingle may have disliked math as a child but then she grew up gravitating toward education, and one thing led to another that turned her into a math teacher. Over her career she taught math to both third and sixth graders in Chattanooga but not -- absolutely not -- the way the nuns taught her. She's retired now, but in the end she was not even teaching the same way she did 30 years ago. A lot has changed. She says she spent a great deal more time trying to help her students understand why they were learning this math. What's it good for? Why does it work? More than anything else, she worked to decrease, if not outright eliminate, the pressure math puts on kids when they don't understand it. It's no joke, this pressure. Like a special freak-out bug that infects math classes. Or as Alice put it, *there's just something weird about math.*

"I'm talking multiplication and division," she told me. "I'm talking decimals. Kids don't know where to put that damn decimal point. And, good grief, don't even talk to me about fractions. Math," she added, "is that subject where everybody stresses out the most. You don't hear about kids stressing out over history."

Alice relied on an ever-increasing number of techniques specifically designed to help get kids comfortable in math world. Her students balanced checkbooks, they played math games, they worked with partners, and they made their numbers mean something. "My students never multiplied 7 times 5 without first giving an example of what those numbers might stand for, like seven groups of 5 animals. Tickets worth $5 to buy for 7 friends."

Sharon Rasch, who teaches math at a public high school here in Knoxville, told me pretty much the same thing. *I don't want these kids to go through what I went through,* she said. Sharon uses the way she was taught as a model for how NOT to teach. "I grew up in the era of memorize-skills-and-do-them, and if you failed, then that door was closed, and you felt terrible, and you said *I suck at math,* while the successful kids were saying *this is so easy, what's wrong with you?* So the strategy has shifted. Problems aren't *problems,* they're tasks tackled by groups of students who begin by coming up with strategies. What's your strategy for starting this task? What's the strategy for completing it? Is it too hard? Let's break it down and look at it again. Not all of it, just this one part. Now, what's the new strategy? Can we model it somehow? Can we draw it, can we visually represent it, can we talk about it so it's not just abstract? What does 4 times 6 mean, really? Four teams of six players. Six apples in four baskets. Four pieces in six chocolate bars. Anything that demonstrates *how* multiplication works. And *why* multiplication works. That's when you're going to get an *ah ha* moment. The entire enterprise is becoming more process focused than answer focused. It's designed to catch a kid before she says, *I'm no good at this.*"

One afternoon I drove out to Nature's Way Montessori School, where my sons went through eighth grade. I admit to the biased belief that Montessori skews the field and pretty much kicks ass when it comes to math, partly because of the Montessori materials. Lower elementary teacher Julie Wolf had arranged for three groups of kids to teach me a variety of lessons, starting with a wooden frame that held strings of colored beads. Two girls showed me how to work it and, watching them, it became clear that concepts like carrying and borrowing are not processes presented like tricks to memorize, but logical conclusions to fooling around with those beads. Who knows if those particular girls will continue to be good math students, but I could see by the way they manipulated the beads how the materials gave them a firm grip on a variety of concepts. Like place value.

My friend Mary Smith owns the school and has taught math to upper elementary students for more than 30 years. She handed me a wooden puzzle with pieces designed to show a trapezoid with an area equivalent to a rectangle next to it. It was unmistakable. The pieces in one fit exactly into the shape of the other. Mary then asked me to come up with the formula to calculate the area of that trapezoid. I had to know a couple of things first, like what equivalent means and that the area of a rectangle is height times the length of its base, which I did know, and which every Montessori student would know before being given this problem to solve. It wasn't easy, honestly, and I felt myself fighting a flutter of panic that I would not be smart enough to figure this out. But playing around with the puzzle pieces, I arrived at the formula all by myself: the area of a trapezoid is $1/2h(b1 + b2)$, where h is height and b is the base.

I know. It's like a goddamned foreign language. But it totally made sense when I saw it laid out in front of me so that I could literally trace the edges of the height and base with my finger. It's almost unfair how helpful these Montessori materials can be.

But I am left with questions. Ms. Tyler, Ms. Ingle, Ms. Rasch, Ms. Wolf, Ms. Smith: great teachers, all of them. Superstars. If I'd had any one of them instead of Mrs. Atwater, would I have been better at math? Would I have remembered more? Would I have had the confidence to take calculus, after all?

On the other hand, all those folks who did love math, was it the particular make-up of their brains that created an opening for a teacher to reach them, or did a particular teacher create the opening? Would they have found a way to love it anyway?

How much does the teaching matter, really?

Here's what I think I know. There's no version of this world in which I would have grown up to be a math major. And yet I do believe I might have missed something important when I was in school. A strong sense of what a number is, for instance. Anything that might have helped me understand that one simple idea might have made a difference. Anything that might have offered me a broader understanding of what math is and more than one way to solve a problem. When there's just one way, you're on a tightrope with a long way to fall.

I don't know how worried to be. The lessons on how to work percentage problems made sense at the time. The logic was evident. We're talking parts of a hundred here, that's all. Who could not see how 30 percent is the same as .30 and also 30/100? Percentage problems looked simple and straightforward, no formulas or tricks, and I remember checking percentages off my list. Fractions, *check*. Decimals, *check*. Percentages *check*. This math business isn't so hard! Time to move on, ever upward.

There is, however, a problem with moving on and ever upward in math. You can't do it. It matters not how many lessons you finish or how much progress you think you've made, you've got to *own* those basic skills you learned, or thought you learned, a long time ago. Own them. Like you don't have to bone up on how to separate eggs before making a cake. Mastery is what the math teachers call it. And bringing students up to mastery turns out to be what elementary school teachers work toward. A kid who masters a concept has a chance to fall in love with math or, at the least, have the tools to be a successful math student. I have been thinking about this, about teachers and what all they are expected to do: how do you teach to mastery when some kids take months to learn what other kids learn in a week? It makes my head hurt to think about it. It makes me want to pay teachers about a million times more than what they make now.

So wait, did I not check percentages off my list? Yes, I did, and yet here I am, staring at a problem and I don't remember what to do.

You go to the store and buy a shirt that ordinarily sells for $75, but today the shirt is marked down 30 percent. How much do you pay? The answer is not 30 percent of 75, which is $22.50, by the way. It's $22.50 *subtracted* from $75. So the answer is $52.50.

I KNOW!

Or I don't know. Or I thought I knew but maybe not? Or sometimes I know but then other times I don't. Or I get in a hurry or I just forget.

The first time I worked the problem, I was nearly drunk with pride to be a person who can take 30 percent of 75, and with brazen confidence I wrote down $22.50, anticipating the exhilaration fueled by a right answer. It's like a sugar hit. There must be something deep and old that lights up when you get a right answer. *You are a good girl. You are a winner. You are confirmed, accepted, loved.*

I check the answer.

The flip side to a right answer is like a physical blow. *You are worthless. Stupid. A loser.* Why is it I can't keep straight so simple a problem as a shirt on sale? The failure goes on forever and never seems to end.

Most of my mistakes are careless errors. It's just so damn easy to add wrong. Once I misread 5 x 4 as 5 x 3. Another time I *added* 2 and 3 when I was supposed to be multiplying. Mistakes like that infuriate me and I want to scream: It's not the *math*, it's the *arithmetic*!

That was me, Miss Righteous Warrior, in math class pretty much all the time. Was it too much to ask that somebody recognize the difference between comprehension mistakes and careless errors? But in math, of course, wrong is wrong. There is no half wrong. And that's a problem for a person who tends to be careless, like me. Like getting a C on an otherwise A+ essay because of spelling.

I actually did once have a teacher, Mrs. Stein, in AP English class my senior year in high school, who gave two grades on every paper, one for content, the other for grammar and, no surprise, I often got that A+/C and felt vindicated. Finally, somebody appreciated what I had to say more than the fact that I misused a comma or two. Or three. For a very long time I wished I could have been similarly graded in math class: *A+ for the algebra, C for that teeny tiny mistake in arithmetic.* Now I'm not so sure.

Those excellent content grades on my essays gave me license to dismiss grammar as unimportant even though it actually is important -- extremely important -- a lesson I had to learn eventually. Might I have been better served had I been held to stricter standards?

And yet those red X's splattered across my math papers weren't good for me, either. They stuck with me as verdicts. Judgments on my character. Where is the line between the number of mistakes it takes to inspire you to do better, and the number that defeats you?

My sons did not make mistakes; they made remedies. At their Montessori school, getting the wrong answer to a problem meant they had to do the problem over again. That was the remedy. Work until you get the right answer. The point was to learn the damn stuff for real, not to be judged on how much one did or did not know at any given point in time. And until they left Nature's Way for public high school, they never got a letter grade on a report card. Day to day they knew how they were doing by how much progress they were making, and they received periodic written evaluations, but their performance was not reduced to a single letter. What even is an A in third grade when working to the top of one's ability differs from kid to kid? What does being labeled a "C" do to a child who's working as hard as possible just to get through a set of 20 division problems?

I'm willing to bet my kids were good at math because, like their father, they were born that way, but I'd toss in a couple of extra bucks on the belief that their school helped. It comes down to a subtle shift in thinking. A remedy can be a helpful indicator of what you need to work on. A mistake can be a red mark on your intelligence. My kids did not carry around the baggage of thinking something might be wrong with them if they messed up on a math test.

Evidently this thinking shift is kind of a big deal in education right now, and it goes by a name: growth mindset. As opposed to fixed mindset. It has roots in research on neuroplasticity and the work of Stanford University psychologist Dr. Carol Dweck, who has studied differences between people who believe what we call our abilities – our talents, capabilities, strengths, skills -- are set in stone, and those who believe those things can be cultivated. I'm simplifying here, but I think of it as the difference between a brain that thinks it was born with an ordained script versus a brain primed to improvise. Evidently, the capacity for brains to change is a relatively new discovery but, regardless, if you don't think your brain can change, then capacity is irrelevant.

A math student with a fixed mindset might say something like: *I don't have a math brain so why bother trying?*

A person with a growth mindset doesn't know the meaning of a math brain and might say something like: *The fact that I didn't do well on this particular test tells me I have to work harder to learn prime factorization but that doesn't mean I'm not good at math. I rock at decimals!*

Or something like that. A fixed mindset can cross generations. Sharon Rasch, who teaches high school algebra and geometry, tells the story of a mother who told her, "My kid's not going to be any good at geometry because I'm terrible at math and I hate math and she's just like me." Teaching is a second career for Sharon, and she was prepared to be challenged by the task of teaching math to students who might or might not be thrilled to learn it. Never once had she anticipated roadblocks placed by a student's own mother.

"The woman said this in front of the kid," Sharon told me, "so now that student is empowered not to do well. As a teacher, where are you then? It's an uphill battle."

It's hard to learn something you've already decided you can't learn.

Math teachers will differ, sometimes dramatically, on fundamental ideas such as which curriculum works best, and I worried initially about getting caught up in arguments such as how do kids really learn? Is a spiral curriculum the way to go? What about those iPads? Hands on materials? How much drilling is too much – how much is not enough? I wondered if I would have to develop an opinion on who was right and who was wrong. But the more I listened, the more I came to understand: none of these teachers uses just one tool, one curriculum, one philosophy, one methodology. Rather, they teach on the assumption that the more lines you toss out, the more fish you'll catch. And every single one of these teachers works to create classroom cultures that encourage the growth mindset.

If you've got a growth mindset, it means you don't think you are smart at math or bad at math or anything. You're just you with a flexible brain capable of learning. You may need a little more time than Susie over there, but she's not necessarily smarter than you are. Mistakes are teaching tools. Embrace them. Learn from them. That goes for math and maybe, I don't know, everything else your whole damn life.

2(5x2) - 11

It's November. We have come to the beach with my parents, to Kiawah Island, South Carolina, the favorite beach when our kids were little, the one we returned to summer after summer, but now the kids have grown up, moved away, and started careers and families of their own, and so summer vacation doesn't mean what it used to mean. When Bruce and I make it back to Kiawah these days it's generally in the fall or winter when the prices go down. This is our first trip to the beach since my mother was diagnosed with Alzheimer's disease, in fact, that's why we're here. It's the first of many trips that I will come to think of as my father's grand project -- to change up my mother's routine, to keep her brain engaged, and to fill the last years of her life, however many that might be, with family.

My father is a man who looks at a problem, seeks to understand it, then attempts to solve it. He is a solver of problems and a man of many projects. I have never seen him bored. I can't even imagine it. If my dad spends any time complaining or bemoaning my mother's

Alzheimer's or wishing it would go away, I have not seen it. He does not talk about it in those terms. We work with what's in front of us, we do what we can. Days after my mother was diagnosed, my father set up an appointment with a woman at the Alzheimer's Association in Chattanooga. The appointment was on a Friday morning in July. I went too.

The woman was nice enough. Right from the get-go I noticed she was making a point to include Mother in the conversation, which we appreciated. Nobody wants anybody treating my mother like a child. "And how do you feel about all this?" the woman asked, and my mother was able to articulate exactly the irony of the disease: she feels fine. It's everybody else who's got the symptoms.

In other words, it's our problem, not hers.

The woman was intent on making sure we understood: Mother won't get better. She might or might not get worse any time soon but there would be no reversal. What capacity she'd already lost, she'd lost, like a penny dropped through a crack in an old porch. You'll never see it again. No cure, no going back, the woman kept repeating it as if used to sitting across the table from people who demand to know how to fix this.

But we weren't those people. We didn't need to be told. We were asking only for guidance, expecting specific information about the disease: stages, symptoms, tips, coping strategies, a booklet, a pamphlet, something. The woman had no pamphlets. Or if she did, she did not offer them to us. Instead, she recommended an Alzheimer's support group. And I thought, fat chance. My parents do not join groups.

To my surprise they did not immediately reject the idea. But the group met in a church in a neighborhood 45 minutes away from their house, so the idea died a natural death from the *no freaking way are we driving all the way out there* argument.

They never joined that group or any group, but my father's mind was open to trying any number of things he might not have considered before. Tai Chi? Probably not, but the stretch class at the club down the street? Maybe. While he ranged around for ideas and options, he was already putting into motion his one sure plan: pack in as much family time as possible. As we were leaving the Alzheimer's Association office, I asked my dad what he wanted to do next. Go to Kiawah, he said.

Alzheimer's is like a lot of things: everybody's different. With my mother, the progression appears to be slow when you look at it day to day, but if you take the perspective of three or four months, the change feels startling.

Is she any worse?

Not really.

Is she worse than she was last summer?

Yes. Absolutely.

Like watching a baby grow, you might not notice the changes as they are happening but every month you've got a different baby. Of course, with a baby you can tick off a lot of what's different. Longer hair, rolling over, sitting up, a tooth, a first word. With my mother, the changes are hard to pin down. I can't come up with an example of this elusive something that's not right and getting more wrong all the time. My dad describes the change in terms of initiative, in the context that Mother doesn't have any. She does not appear to want to do, well, anything. Knowing what you want and how to get it: that's a skill she's losing.

Here I simply have to pause to say, this is my mother we're talking about. Charlotte Elaine Walker Landis, a woman who used to check out the theater section of *The New Yorker*, pick up the phone, buy tickets, make hotel and plane reservations, just like that. Boom. Done. A woman who would drive to Atlanta to see a movie that was not showing in Chattanooga. A woman who started an arts organization for Chattanooga artists because, well, it didn't have one. A woman who could throw a dinner party for 2 or 20, no sweat. Now she can't remember how to make slaw. She can't seem to get off the couch.

What my dad called initiative is also known as executive function. This is how Dr. Lindquist explained it to me. Dr. Lindquist is the Northwestern University gerontologist I talked to one extremely cold Chicago winter morning. After short-term memory, executive function is generally the next thing to go in Alzheimer's. It's tempting to think of losing functions like losing a list of possessions –first you lose your sweater, then your keys, then your shoes, but Dr. Lindquist prefers the analogy of peeling layers of an onion, where one layer is dependent on another. To get from here to there takes steps, she explained. If you can't remember the steps, it's scary.

The day before we are to leave Kiawah, Bruce and I take my mother for a walk on the beach. My dad has stayed behind to work on a jigsaw puzzle. As we approach the boardwalk back to the condominium, Bruce and I decide to keep walking, but Mother is ready to go inside. A flicker of a decision crosses my mind. Before this Alzheimer's business, it never would have occurred to me that I might ought to take her back to the condo. The condo is right there at the end of the boardwalk, for heaven's sake. But I hesitate. Should I go back with her? I don't like treating her like a child. I don't want her to think that I think she could get lost, that she needs to be accommodated, like something is wrong with her.

I get her to the edge of the boardwalk, making sure she's on the one that leads directly back to the condominium. By directly, I mean that it ends at a point where, turning left gets you to our building. You can turn right, but that's another building. Since we've been here, we have never once turned right. You turn left, walk to the elevator, take it up to the second floor, and right there in front of you is our condo. We have taken this path for four days already, back and forth to the beach several times a day. I'm thinking there's no way she can get lost – the condo is *right there*.

Still. Maybe I'm overreacting, but I text my dad, anyway. *Mother's coming up. Look for her.* Then Bruce and I resume our walk. How long were we gone? Hard to tell, maybe 30 minutes? We're busy talking, we walk up the boardwalk, we turn left, we take the stairs up to the second floor and open the door to the condo. My dad is still working on the jigsaw puzzle.

"Where's Mother?"

"I thought she was with you."

His phone is on the dresser in the bedroom. He has not seen my text.

I rush out to find her while Dad and Bruce stay on the balcony outside the door in case she comes back before I do. I search the parking lot as if there might be some hidden spot. Our building is the first of four that look relatively similar, same architecture, same brown cedar shake siding, and when she's clearly nowhere in the parking lot in front of our building, I hurry over to the second one. Then the third and the one beyond that. I'm scouring the parking lots but also the buildings where I can see into the open breezeways on each floor. I am starting to panic. She has to be somewhere, but where?

I see a man working at the far end of the parking lot in front of building number 4, and I run over there. Here, finally, is somebody to ask, *have you seen ...,* but as I'm running, I look up. And there she is. My mother, walking along the breezeway on the second floor, three buildings down from where she's supposed to be.

"Mother!"

She's startled to hear my voice. Is she relieved? I can't tell for sure. She never thought she was lost. At least that's what she says as we walk back. She wasn't *worried*. She would have found the right condo *eventually*, she says.

But she wouldn't have. She didn't just have the wrong building; she was looking for the wrong unit number. And yet she appears less worried about the prospect of being lost than about what Daddy's going to think. She talks about that, a lot, about how much Daddy worries, as if he shouldn't. As if he's making mountains out of molehills. As if Daddy worrying, Daddy taking over the cooking, the driving, the bills, Daddy telling her what to do all the time, is the primary symptom of her disease. She's missing the part where she doesn't remember how to make a pie, or that she's telling me the same thing she told me minutes ago, or that she could not find her way back to the condominium at the beach. She's feeling the disease through the reactions of my father.

My dad is shaken. Me too. You think you sort of know what you're dealing with but how can you? We can't know what she doesn't know. At this point, we can't even predict what she can't do anymore. And yet -- here is evidence of another change. It feels significant. Another layer of the onion. It's hard to keep up with a disease that's so silent and sneaky.

Back at the condo we are laughing, ha, ha, what an adventure. *I wasn't lost!* She says it again. Weren't we silly to worry? She's fine! No big deal. She sits down and looks at my dad.

"Is it too early for vodka?"

So maybe she's worried, after all? I have no idea.

My dad is. It's been months since the last time my mother drove a car, but her keys are still in her purse. When they get home, he takes them out and hides them.

25/5 x 8/4

Consider a plate of cookies. Two-thirds of them are small. Five-sevenths of the small cookies are chocolate. What fraction of the cookies are small and chocolate?

I was feeling confident. I looked at that cookie problem and said, I can do this! So I did it. Multiply 5/7 by 2/3 to get 10/21. It made sense to think of taking a fraction of a fraction of all of the cookies on the plate. Next question.

Three-fifths of the books in the library are non-fiction. One-twelfth of those are biographies. What fraction of the books in the library are biographies?

Same as the cookie problem. Right? Multiply 3/5 by 1/12. But before I could even think about calculating, I got hung up on the BOOKS IN THE LIBRARY part of the problem. To me that meant ALL the books, non-fiction and fiction.

In the cookie problem, I was asked to compute how many of JUST THE SMALL cookies were chocolate, not ALL the cookies. There very well could be 30 large sugar cookies on that plate along with the small chocolate ones but I was not being asked about those. Some of the large cookies also could have been chocolate but I was not being asked about those either. I was being asked to calculate only the fraction of the small cookies that are chocolate.

But in the library problem, I was not being asked to calculate how many of the non-fiction books are biographies. I was supposed to find out how many of ALL the books are biographies, so multiplying the fraction of non-fiction books by the number of biographies made no sense to me. I drew pictures, circles divided into fifths, shading three, and those divided into 12, shading one. Still it made no sense.

I took the problem to Bruce. I've have noticed that he looks at math problems as wholes rather than parts, like he sees an entire field of flowers from the air while I'm picking over weeds. He is also not afraid of math. Bruce tells me to multiply the fraction of non-fiction books by the number of biographies: $3/5 \times 1/12 = 3/60$, which simplifies to $1/20$. So I do it. Maybe it's the right answer.

It is, actually, the right answer.

I still don't get it. I worry I'm overthinking again. What am I missing?

Oranges are 30 percent off but only today. I buy 6 oranges and am charged $12.60. Tomorrow I want to buy 2 more oranges. How much will I have to pay for those two oranges?

Here comes another problem that looks easy to me. My confidence is high, and on this particular morning I am in a groove. Knock this one out and I'll be done with math for the day; that's the plan, only I end up working on it for most of the morning. I mean, I clear the desk, fill pages of yellow legal pad paper with calculations, draw pictures of oranges, sharpen my pencil a half-dozen times, pace. The solution hovers close, but hours later, still no answer. I stop only because I am supposed to meet my friend Lettie for coffee.

I take the problem with me, copied out on a piece of paper. I place it on the table in front of us. Lettie tells me she was good at math in school. Taking one look at the problem, she jumps right in. This is the sort of problem that used to be fun for me, she says.

But Lettie is out of practice. It has been a long time since she's sat down to work an actual math problem. Clearly there is a way to solve it, a simple and logical way, perhaps a trick of some kind, but as with me, the solution hovers just outside her grasp. Her first instinct is to devise a ratio.

It's a good instinct. No question, you can solve this problem with a ratio, although we aren't having any luck. My first instinct was to turn it into an equation. Also a good instinct. We applaud each other's instincts.

In my equation, X would stand for the full price of one orange. $12.60 divided by 6 gives you 2.10, which is the sale price of one orange. With those assumptions, I have come up with:

$X - (.30X) = 2.10$.

Which gets me nowhere. Actually, it gets me to $0 = 70$, the 0 being what happens when you divide both sides by .30, leaving X-X. Lettie is also playing around with 70 in her ratio but it isn't leading her to an answer. When we leave the coffee shop, she vows to keep trying. I text my son Charlie.

Charlie texts back with the answer in less than a minute. Problem solved. One regular priced orange is $3. *Seems pretty expensive,* he adds.

How did he do it?

He writes back: *$12.60 divided by 6 is $2.10. $2.10 is 70 percent of $3.00, which I got by dividing $2.10 by 7 and then multiplying by 10. That means 30 percent off of $3.00 is $2.10.*

Um. So how did he know how to do that?

I dunno, he writes. *It's just a trick I use automatically with percentages. Simplifying your terms is generally a good first step I think.*

Yes, I write him back, but I would still have to fall back on some sort of standard tool, like an equation or ratio. I don't know how I would ever have gotten to your original solution.

My original solution isn't algebra, though, he writes. *It's just a method my brain has devised for dealing with problems like this in my head.*

His brain. Okay, I tell him, I think your brain has a much more organic relationship with numbers and what they symbolize. So you can make some leaps in your mind that I can't make.

Perhaps, says Charlie. *You still might benefit from my rule of thumb. If there's a calculation that's too tricky to do by itself, try to break it up into smaller parts. Like, I can't automatically divide 2.10 by 0.7 but I can't understand that 2.10 is seven tenths of the answer I'm looking for, so I can find one tenth by dividing by 7 and then finding the whole by multiplying by 10. It's easier in parts like that.*

Got that?

Me neither.

But he did point out the mistake I made in my equation. X is actually 1X. Of course. And so to return: X − (.30X) = 2.10. I should have subtracted first. 1X - .30X = 2.10, which simplifies to .7X − 2.10, which gives me 3.

Lettie got to 3, too. Very quickly, it turns out, as soon as she sat down at her desk in her quiet office where she could think. She called to tell me. Relieved. It is unnerving to believe you know how to do a simple thing only to have it elude you, I understand that. I am happy she is relieved, but I am still unnerved.

I have set out to learn, or relearn, enough math so I am no longer innumerate. And while I'd like to go further, I am wondering if there are limits. I'm confident of it, actually. Where the limits are, I don't know, only that there are places in math I cannot go. Some brains are better at this stuff than other brains. They just are.

99/9

My mother and I used to talk, if not every day, then almost. Our talks could run up to an hour, quite a chunk of time when you're busy, but I don't remember ever regretting the time. Sometimes talking to my mother was the best part of my day. When I was a new mother, full of doubt and worry and fear and loneliness, conversations with my mother saved my life.

What did we talk about? Everything. Books, music, food, art, friends, kids, politics, religion, and my mother's clothes. We recommended articles for each other to read, recipes to try, movies to see. My mother was an engaging and entertaining woman, interesting, sharp, well read, curious, and really, really funny. She was one of the "cool moms" when I was in high school, not because she wasn't strict – she could be pretty damn strict and sometimes arbitrarily so – but nobody else's mom was listening to Aretha Franklin and James Brown. She was the first mom to switch to whole wheat bread, which might sound like a silly thing to remember but in those white bread times, whole wheat was a cultural signal of progressive environmental consciousness. She moved us from the First Christian Church to St. Paul's Episcopal because, among other reasons, that's where the liberal people went. In what was considered a bold move, she went back to college for a second degree when I was 16. My mother was a woman on the move. She was change. A forward thinker. A never-settler. This made her the ideal mother for a teenager like me.

My mother was 24 when I was born. Probably too young, but she had only a vague sense of that. She'll admit she didn't know what she was doing. She knew what the books told her, and the books told her to get those babies on a schedule. She could be kind and fun and generous but I suspect she approached raising my brother and me as a job with rules she was required to follow. It would not have occurred to her that we could just as well eat broccoli, which we liked, instead of the slimy okra, which we hated, and we wouldn't end up with scurvy or grow up to be juvenile delinquents. To her, the okra was on the table, the okra was what she'd cooked us, and by golly we were going to sit there until we ate it. That was my mother when I was a child. But as I grew, she grew, and she grew into a mother who listened to me. I can think of no greater gift.

I mark the birth of my first son as the moment when our relationship made it's definitive shift from mother/daughter to something closer to friendship. My son Bruce Jr. was born in August, two months after my husband Bruce and I moved to Augusta, Georgia, where he started a fellowship in pulmonary medicine and where I knew no one. No friends, no job, no money. I'd never been around a baby before, had never once even changed a diaper. If Bruce could have stayed home those first weeks we could have made it without my mother, but he was working all the time. She came and stayed for two weeks, taking care of me while I learned how to take care of the baby. When she left, we worked out a system for talking on the phone. Long distance phone calls were expensive, and we had no money, and so when I wanted to talk, I'd call her, let it ring once, then hang-up. That was the signal for her to call me back, which meant she paid for all of our conversations. As a new mother with no friends in Augusta, Georgia, I was in the wilderness. She was my lifeline.

In time she became my best editor. Writers need readers, and sometimes you can count on friends or fellow-writers for that, but friends and fellow writers are not always brutally honest. They will hedge. They will tolerate a certain measure of bullshit. Some give more weight to sentence structure than plot coherence, while for others it's just the opposite. Through my many years of unpublished short stories to my first published novel and the novels that came after that, my mother was not merely willing to listen to the struggles and triumphs (mostly struggles) of my fledgling career, she ended up being the one person I could turn to for no-nonsense, honest, clear-headed, and insightful criticism, and I'm talking sentence structure, plot coherence, character development, and spelling.

Writing that last sentence, I have had to stop. I'm sitting in my kitchen in front of my computer, staring at the screen, realizing that she can't be my editor anymore. Realizing this very book is the first piece of writing I've ever attempted without her feedback. My mother was my one reader who did not let me get away with any-thing -- not sloppy writing, not sloppy thinking, and I counted on it. I didn't necessarily agree with every suggestion she offered, but each one forced me to think. She made me a better writer.

Now what?

For a while, I continued to send her drafts because she could still correct my spelling, and it maintained at least the trappings of our old relationship, but she appears to have lost the ability to read critically. She's missing nuance. And like so many aspects of this frustrating disease, I can't pinpoint a time when she stopped being able to think the way she used to. I can't pinpoint the moment our talks began to change.

I want to. Irrationally, and futilely, I keep coming back to the same questions: when did I first notice something was off? Were there signs two years ago? Three years ago? I ask knowing that an answer solves nothing, proves nothing, suggests nothing, and yet I keep asking. It's like half of me wants to grow up and accept this disease while the other half is jumping up and down, yelling, *What is happening! When did this shit begin! Why can't I talk to my mother?*

Of course, we do talk, still. But I make allowances for what she can and can't remember. I accommodate for the fact that she doesn't do anything anymore. There are no more meetings to tell me about. No decisions or controversies. She's not following the news. She's not keeping up with the movies. If she's read any books lately, she's lost the capacity to talk about them. She isn't planning any more parties. She isn't buying new clothes. Mainly what we talk about these days are the weather, her dog, and how lucky she and Daddy are to have their health. Her memories are softer, tending more toward funny moments that happened when she was younger. Each time we talk I'm prepared to respond to things she's already told me as if I've never heard them before. Measuring my words, limiting their scope and depth, monitoring my tone for any hint of impatience. It's not like talking to my mother. It's not unlike talking to a child.

It's hard for me not to think of math as a race where you beat one level then move on to the next and then the next. After the basics – adding, subtracting, multiplying, dividing -- come fractions, decimals, percentages, ratios and proportions, negative numbers, exponents, square roots, graphing, prime numbers, algebra, geometry, algebra II, trigonometry, statistics, and then calculus. More or less. It's a rough sequence I have stuck in my mind, and it spurs me to climb ever higher, never falling back. I don't know why falling back feels like a kind of failure but it does. It *seems* as if I should be able to learn something once and then not have to learn it again, but that's not happening. I tell myself to calm down. The problem is very likely a matter of practice, which I continue to underestimate because I'm in a hurry, in a race to get to the next level. But it is, simply, impossible to get around the fact that a couple of lessons on percentages six weeks ago is not enough. If I were in fifth grade,

I'd be spending weeks on percentage problems. I'd be percentigizing the heck out of shirts and fruit and gumballs and sports teams, and then I'd do it again in sixth grade, and if I kept with it, working out percentages throughout my math class trajectory and on into life outside of school, so that maybe by now it would be as central to my core expertise as is knowing a stick of butter is a half a cup. Practice is called for. Practice is essential. There are no short cuts.

A pile of workbooks sits on a dining room chair. I see them every time I walk through the room. I hide them when I have friends over because this innumeracy is still hard to admit. The workbooks represent what I should know already, mocking me for what I should have learned this second go-round.

But when, and if, I remember – there is no time clock, no finish line -- I can force myself to stop moving forward. I stop and pick up one of the workbooks and sit down and practice. Forty pages of fundamentals. This stuff has to become second nature, like riding a bike, driving a car, writing this sentence. What shame can there be in slowing down? No one cares how fast I learn this math. No one cares if I ever do. I'm just hoping practice is the reason I'm slow and not that something's wrong with my brain.

Are some people prone to careless errors? Yes. Mary Smith at Nature's Way Montessori says it comes down to attention and focus. Focused kids are thinking about what they are doing when they are doing it and so they are less likely to mistake 2 x 3 for 2 + 3.

I am not focused. My husband Bruce is focused. So are our sons. More than once I've caught all three of those guys thinking about what they are doing when they are doing it. My mind is ever in a million places. I am sloppy, the opposite of attentive and intentional. In my house, you might come across doors left open, but I won't have noticed. Shoes are scattered all over the place. Watching me chop vegetables, you might find it stunning that I still have 10 fingers. I have no idea how I manage to drive a car. I don't know why I'm not dead yet.

In an attempt to compensate, I have begun writing everything down when I work math problems, and it seems to help, a little. I copy every single problem out on a piece of paper with a pencil before trying to solve it. Even simple parts: like if I'm supposed to take half of 10. It's 5, I know it's 5, of course it's 5, but if I take the time to write down: $10/ 2 = 5$, I make fewer mistakes. I hate it. But I do it anyway. As much as I want to believe I can handle a few quick calculations in my head, shortcuts leave too much room for mistakes. And when I work in this careful way, *if* I will work in this careful way, math slows me down. It forces me take one step at a time. That's focus. Right?

Still. What if something else is going on? Because I sense it. I've always been sloppy, but these days my brain seems to be working more slowly than it used to. Like the time between the beginning of a thought and the end is getting longer. Like sentences dropped halfway through are getting more frequent. Like the tendency to flit around from thought to thought is getting harder to corral. It's a cliché to say something is "gumming up" the parts up there, but that's what it feels like. Unless I'm being fooled by suggestive thinking. When you spend a lot of time thinking about Alzheimer's, it's hard not to look for signs.

It is possible that I personally, already focus-challenged, have become more susceptible to that mind-stealing monster, distraction. And as embarrassing as my math deficits might be, it feels worse somehow to be easily distractible. Like in a hierarchy of weaknesses, distraction is more damning than innumeracy. Distraction makes me picture an eight-year-old boy who can't sit still, not a 60-year-old grandmother. Admittedly, spending hours on this computer to write this book has not helped, with the emails beckoning to be checked and today's news and bank statements and calendars and recipes, followed by an urgent need to make more granola or the lure of a half-finished podcast. It feels ironic that I have picked a cultural moment of such enormous distraction to venture on this quest to become more focused.

I suspect the more distracted you become, the slower your mind works, and the slower your mind works, the more susceptible to distraction it becomes, and so it's a loop. It's hard to break out of a loop. If succumbing to distractions has changed my brain like water carving out ever-deepening gullies, then it might not be too late to reverse the damage, to heal a bit, to change my habits and thereby change my brain. But if my actual brain is not as resilient as it was when it was younger, not as strong, not as disciplined, then my increased distractibility is a symptom of a much bigger problem. My hair is graying. My skin is thinning. Is my brain slowing down?

I have read that even healthy brains shrink by roughly 10 percent between the ages of 50 and 80. Ten years down that road already, I have to ask, does it matter? Is brain size destiny? Can I fight this? Evidently it has been established that you can combat aging's inevitable loss of balance with yoga. The inevitable loss of muscle mass with weights. So here's a question: if I can figure out how to decrease distraction, will my brain work better? I have to try. Meditation, that's supposed to help. Untethering from the internet, that's another thing that's supposed to help. Sleep. Exercise. And math?

Here's an equation: how many math problems does it take to counter one glass of wine.

(4 x 3) + 1

Runner A runs 15 miles per week. If she adds 1 mile per week, how long before she can run 13.6 miles in a day?

The half marathon I trained for is in Chattanooga on a Sunday morning in October. The night before the race, my father has cooked pasta and shrimp. Over dinner we talk about breakfast, which will have to be fast and easy since I need to leave the house by 5:45. I decide on hardboiled eggs and a granola bar. After dinner I put some water on to boil and drop in a couple of eggs.

One thing about my mother's memory: it's inconsistent. She can know I'm in town to run a half-marathon but cannot remember what we just talked about

"Should we put on some eggs to boil?" she asks as we are finishing the dishes.

I point to the eggs in the pot of boiling water.

Dishes washed, eggs cooked and cooling in the refrigerator, we move to the living room.

"What do you want to do for breakfast?" she asks.

"I think I'll have a hardboiled egg and a granola bar," I say, cheerfully.

"Should we boil the eggs?"

"Already done it. No worries."

Twenty minutes later: "What do you want to do for breakfast?"

I count 5 times she asks, not that counting matters. After the fifth time, I catch my dad shooting me a look as if to say, *are you hearing this?*

Loud and clear. Later that night I ask him. "She's getting worse, isn't she?"

"Yes."

Alzheimer's disease affects 47 million people worldwide, a number that's growing fast. By 2050 it's expected to hit 135 million and will kill more people than cancer. A brain with Alzheimer's is not the same as an old brain. It's a brain under attack. It's a brain experiencing catastrophic nerve cell death, but nobody seems to know for certain what causes it or how to stop it. There are clues, lots of clues and theories, and a bunch of research chasing down every hunch, but nothing so definitive as to be free of detractors.

One leading theory is known as the amyloid cascade hypothesis, which asserts that the formation of beta-amyloid plaques could cause the disease. Beta-amyloid is not a virus or bacteria or any other outside agent, but, rather, a part of our brains. Naturally. Evidently, we don't know exactly what it is. It looks like a protein that works on the surface of neuron cells, assisting with communication or protection or something benign and supportive. But when malfunctioning fragments of this stuff drift away from the cells, they stick together with other fragments to form plaques that grow until eventually they block the neurons from chemicals that are necessary for their survival. Basically, the cells kill themselves. This plaque-forming process can start early, as early as when you're 40 or 50 years old, but may take decades to produce symptoms. Like suicide bombers waiting for a sign.

But that's just a theory, and there are other theories, focusing on different aspects peculiar to the disease such as tangles that form inside neurons, genetic mutations, and a runaway immune response. There are no definitive answers on what causes the disease: genes, environmental toxins, lifestyle, bad luck, all of the above, or none of the above. And recent studies have been undermining the amyloid hypothesis all together. Autopsies have revealed plaque-filled brains in people with no symptoms. Conversely, some people die of Alzheimer's with brains that show up entirely disease-free. So many questions!

Alzheimer's may not be one single disease. Alzheimer's may not always be Alzheimer's. Patients diagnosed with Alzheimer's might have experienced silent strokes, or dementia caused by unrelated proteins, or by who knows what. It may be less a disease than a process. It makes me think of cancer, in that the body might be turning on itself, only worse because at least some cancers can be cured. There's no cure for Alzheimer's, not yet. No surgery, no chemo, no radiation, no medication. You can't go to a therapist and talk your way out of this one. Some researchers argue that we are decades from finding a cure, which makes it imperative that we study ways to help patients live in dignity with the disease throughout all its phases.

I am considering my mother's brain. As I listen to her talk, I imagine it filled with tangled gray masses, like steel wool, some patches thicker and darker than others, through which light flashes intermittently. Talking to her feels like watching one of those flashes strike, lighting up a specific bundle of thoughts. For the time being, the light is on breakfast, but that will pass. When a different subject – let's say her brother Raymond -- lights up, Mother knows exactly what to say as if there's an envelope containing a finite number of things to say about him, which she pulls out, one by one. The light flashes, the envelope opens, and she ticks through the contents as if for the first time. No recollection that she's said any of these things many, many times before. She might even do it more than once, telling me the same Raymond story she just told me. But eventually the light goes out until the next time Raymond's name comes up. The same is true for most of what she talks about to the point where I can predict what she's going to say about most every subject. From what I can tell, my mother is not originating new thoughts.

Of course, I cannot know what's happening inside my mother's brain. All I have to go on is what she says and does. She is confused, more and more so. Packing for a trip out to California to see my brother, she has to ask my dad more than once: *Where are we going?* And there's this shuffle walk she does now, her feet splayed outward. It is not my mother's walk. And there's a quality to her voice that I can't quite put my finger on, a timbre that doesn't sound like her. Hesitant, but more than that. Lost. It's like she's searching for words, but not just words. Searching.

Or am I imagining this searching? How can I know? I can't know. I can't ask, and she can't tell me. This is what I'm thinking about on the afternoon after my half-marathon, sitting on the porch with my mother, who is telling me a story about her brother that I have heard more times than I can count. It is a sunny autumn afternoon and I am feeling a little lost, myself.

My time for the race was two hours and twenty minutes. It's not a great time, but apparently it's not bad for an amateur of my age.

We had trained for it. By *we*, I mean my running partners Teri and her brother Brent. Together we had run through some hot summer months including one memorable windless August morning when I did not bring enough water for an 11-mile run but I ran it anyway and almost passed out before reaching my car. This is the sort of reckless behavior you expect from a 20-year-old, not so much a 60-year-old grandmother. Where are the lines: between aging with grace and surrender, between defiance and acceptance, between courage and foolishness, between perseverance and delusion. Why do I run? Some of the reasons are healthy.

The race itself was hard. Harder than I'd expected given all that training. Twice we'd run twelve miles. You would think running 13 would not be so much different from running 12. Wouldn't you? Just one more mile?

Race-day adrenaline both drove me and wore me out. It was dark still when we got to the park where the race began but the place was lit up like a party. Some radio station was pumping out dance music. We were jumping up and down with thousands of people, stretching our quads, our hamstrings, our calves, our Achilles tendons. Going to the bathroom *one more time.* Thousands of people. Some of them would run the full marathon, crossing the Tennessee River seven times, befitting the name: Seven Bridges Marathon. For the half, we would cross four times. I ran across the Market Street Bridge as the sun was coming up. By mile three, already I was thinking, *I can't do this.*

Mile 6 brought a tingling sensation to my left foot that did not speak well for at least one of my nerves. Mile 10 reminded me that my hips had never agreed to this bone-headed adventure. I was hobble-running, gritting teeth, counting: *if you can run 10, you can run 11, then 12, then ...* Mile 13 was a whirlwind, a rush, a dream. Until I stopped running and then could hardly walk.

Honestly, I was glad it was hard. Relieved, actually, limping around in my stiffening body. Because I know how I can get sometimes, and if 13 had been easy, I would have begun romanticizing 26.

None of that surprised me. Nerve pain, hip pain, adrenaline surges all fell into a category of possible things that can happen to you when you get up before dawn to run 13 miles with thousands of other people. The surprise came later. Not in the park with the rousing dance music and boisterous crowd and vendors in booths handing out granola bars and energy drinks, but in the leaving. It was time to leave but I did not want to. I almost didn't know how.

I'd done it!

Sixty-year-old me trained to run 13 miles, ran 13 miles, celebrated the running of the 13 miles, but eventually there was nothing more to do but turn and walk across one more bridge toward the parking garage where I had to get in the car and drive away.

Now what.

(4 x 5) - 6

Two trains leave the station from different cities heading toward each other at different speeds. Train A, traveling at 70 mph, leaves East Town heading toward West Town, 260 miles away. At the same time, Train B, traveling 60 mph, leaves West Town heading toward East Town. How long will it take for the two trains meet?

It's kind of like a joke, the two trains problem. I mean, I have only to say -- *two trains* -- and people know I'm talking about math. It's like a code. Like the magic words for mental time travel, taking them back to some distant classroom in some school where they are sitting at a desk working word problems. Even people who are good at math, who remember how to work two trains problems and can pick up pencil and paper and solve one right this minute, understand the joke. It's like kale. Some people love kale. I'm one of those people, but I understand that it's a punchline to connote foods you might not want at a birthday party. I'm tired of the joke of the two trains. I want to get serious about this word problem business. I've been working on math for a while now, and I am ready to be a person who can solve this damn problem.

There is a formula. It helps if you know the formula. The formula is, Distance equals Speed times Time, which you can write as: $D = S(T)$. You can switch it around so it goes, Speed equals Distance divided by Time, or: $S = D/T$. Some people say rate instead of speed – no problem, then it's just $D = R(T)$ or $R = D/T$. With such a formula, you ought to be able to plug those numbers in and calculate your way to an answer. Right?

So I do that. Distance is 260, but speed? I'm looking at two speeds here -- 70 mph and 60 mph. What am I supposed to do with two speeds? The formula doesn't say anything about two speeds!

I have the answer right here in front of me underneath a picture of a tiny blue train on its tiny track and a tiny red train on its tiny track. Speed, as it turns out for this problem, is 70 + 60. So the equation looks like this: $260 = 70(T) + 60(T)$, or $260 = 130(T)$. Divide both sides by 130 and you get $T=2$. So it's 2. The answer is 2. The two trains will meet each other in two hours. Great.

But how was I supposed to know to *add* the 70 and the 60?

There is nothing in that formula that signals *addition*, and my heart is speeding up, and I can almost feel myself back in eighth grade, watching Mrs. Haskins show us how to work the problem on the blackboard, and I'm just supposed to memorize how to do it so I can – *what*? Get my homework done and make a good grade on a test? How does that help me? It doesn't help me. It doesn't tell me why. WHY does it work? WHY?

I'm getting mad just thinking about it.

I show the problem to Bruce. If one train is going in one direction, he says, and the other in the opposite direction, at different speeds, one will get to the mid-point faster than the other, and so, he concludes, the question is about time. Then he starts talking about relative speed. He talks about what it would seem like, riding in the blue train, watching the world go by at 70 miles an hour, when suddenly a 60 mile-an-hour red train whooshes past *way* faster than the trees and houses and cows you've been passing – most likely at a rate of something like 60 + 70.

Is he trying to tell me that I have to understand the concept of relative speed before I can solve this stupid problem?

Bruce solves the problem, but I'm so agitated and impatient by now I start emailing other people to help. Then I worry that I've panicked too soon. Am I doing this to myself? Churning somewhere underneath my consciousness is a sense of self-sabotage, like I'm throwing obstacles in front of myself that keep me from solving these math problem. What obstacles? I have no idea. It's just a sense I have, a suspicion I cannot identify or articulate, some inkling that I'm not giving myself a chance. But how do you clear out an obstacle if you don't know what the obstacle is?

I stare at the picture of the tiny green train and the tiny red train on their tiny tracks, and I study the solution to the problem below the picture, and if I squint really hard I can almost see that it might make sense to add.

Soon friends come through with the solution to the problem – it's 2. Right. Two hours, got it. But they all got there in different ways.

My math professor friend Carl sent this:
After t hours, train A will have covered 60t miles, and train B, 70t miles, for a total of 130t miles. When 130t =260, i.e., when t=2, the trains meet.

My friend Grier sent this:

rA = 70 mph
rB = 60 mph
d=rt
t = tA = tB
dA + dB = 260
rAtA + rBtB = 260
rAt + rBt = 260
70t + 60t = 260
130t = 260
t = 260/130
t = 2

My son Charlie sent this:

I think it helps to take it hour by hour. After one hour, train A will have traveled 70 miles and train B will have traveled 60 miles, knocking 130 miles off the total distance. That leaves 130 miles remaining, so in another hour, the trains will meet. Does that make sense?

Yes. I think it does. Maybe.

Ernest Hemingway said the trick to writing is you sit down and write one sentence and then you write another one and then you write another one. By *writing*, he wasn't talking about the happy scribbling away of a writer who can't get the words down fast enough; in fact, just the opposite. He was talking about writer's block. Ernest Hemingway was prescribing a cure for writer's block.

Except Hemingway never actually said that. I only *thought* that's what he'd said. I had thought it for a very long time, and for a very long time I summoned those words often when I was in need of a kick in the butt: *Sit down, write a goddamn sentence! Then another and then another.* I used Hemingway's words as desperate inspiration on those days when I was afraid to write. I extrapolated them to apply to any number of things. Running when you want to stop, well, take one more step and then another. Practicing the piano, well, play just the right hand and then the left. Hike one more mile.

Swim one more lap. Make one more phone call. Clean one more closet. Then one day I looked it up.

What Ernest Hemingway actually said, or at least what he is said to have said about writing, is this: *"All you have to do is write one true sentence. Write the truest sentence that you know. So finally I would write one true sentence, and then go on from there."*

What I thought he had said -- compared to what he actually said -- might sound like the same thing, but it isn't. There is a difference between writing one sentence and writing one true sentence. Hemingway was talking less about stamina and persistence and more about precision. Writing is hard work, but it's much, much easier to write something that's not quite true. And by *true*, I don't mean in the sense that grass is green and rocks are hard. It's not about facts that can be proven true or false. It's not about fiction versus nonfiction. It's deeper than that.

You can open a jar of marinara sauce and pour it into a pot and heat it and spread it over pasta. You can also cut up fresh tomatoes and garlic and onions and cook them in olive oil infused with a couple of smashed anchovies over low heat for two hours and spread that over pasta. But there is a difference. I wish it weren't so ridiculously easy to slip into writing something facile, quick, and miles away from genuine. Hollow sentences that don't advance a plot or build an argument, sentences that may be beautiful but float around existing for their own sake. Misfired metaphors, pretty words, tired words, sloppy words, sentiments divorced from emotion. But it is. Easy. So easy that it's difficult to recognize what you're doing. So easy, why try harder?

Here's a sentence that is true: I am working math problems to exercise my brain because some studies suggest that learning new things, particularly hard things, may delay the onset of Alzheimer's disease.

Here's a true sentence: I'm spending tons of time alone, time that I barely have in my busy day, working math problems to exercise my brain on the unproven chance that it will protect me from Alzheimer's, even though I fear it may not be working because already I'm sensing my brain is not as quick as it used to be, like some sort of gears are jamming, so maybe it's too late because whatever's in there jamming the gears is only going to grow and spread, and then what if I end up like my mother, except what if there's nobody who can take care of me by then, and I end up in some horrible institution where I don't even get to pick out what I eat for my own goddamn lunch?

When my mother moved my grandmother into an assisted living facility, I went down there to help. My grandmother was moving from a three-bedroom house into what was essentially a bedroom with a kitchenette tacked on to one end. My grandmother's old house had not been particularly large but she'd lived there almost 50 years and it had a sunroom off the kitchen with lots of windows and a television where she spent most of her time with her sweet, old, blind dog. To move to the assisted living facility, she had to get rid of the dog.

This all happened some 25 years ago, and I had forgotten about the dog until just recently. I can't even remember his name, but there are pictures of my grandmother with her dog, and my parents and I were looking at them as we sorted through old family photographs. We all remembered that day. My parents helped pack up the house, the movers came, and then it was time for my grandmother to say goodbye to the dog. Goodbye in the sense that as soon as my mother drove her away, my father was going to put the dog in his car and drive him to the vet where he would be euthanized. It was horrible. But at the time there appeared to be no other option. My grandmother could no longer care for the dog. Nobody else wanted him, and it was said that it would be cruel to force an old blind dog to learn how to navigate in a new place. It was said that dying was in the dog's best interest. That kind of goodbye.

I wasn't there for the leaving of the dog. By the time I got down to Chattanooga my grandmother was trying to get settled into her new home, or more to the point, her new room. I should say that of all the people I've ever known to live in an assisted living arrangement, my grandmother was the most suited for it. She was a social, extroverted person, and living alone with no ability to drive anywhere was not healthy for her. She ended up thriving in a place where friends and companions lived down the hall, but the first few months were hard. That particular day was especially hard. Trying to make the whole shitty situation seem less shitty, my mother was grasping for positives. Such a nice carpet! Pretty drapes! A small refrigerator *and* a microwave.

Standing in the middle of her new one room, trying to catch the positives my mother was tossing her way, my grandmother appeared lost. Yes, it is a nice carpet and the drapes are pretty, I imagined her thinking, *but surely I'm not going to have to fucking live here?* After an aide popped in to explain how the laundry service worked, my mother exclaimed, "Just think, they even do your laundry!"

My grandmother, smiling because she was supposed to be thrilled by this news, answered, "But what will I do?"

It was almost a whisper. Like she didn't mean to be ungrateful but ...

What will I do?

My heart broke so hard I ended up writing my first novel based on this one moment when an old woman begins to lose her place in the world. If you're in charge of washing the clothes and the clothes don't get washed, somebody notices. It's a job that needs doing. It's important. Instinctively my grandmother longed for a job to do, she wanted to feel important, necessary, noticed. At the least she wanted to do her own laundry. Now what?

How are we to spend our days? Should we long for a state of perpetual vacation where nothing is required, where everything is done for us? Would the best of all possible days allow the freedom to sit around reading, eating, watching TV? With all that freedom would we take up painting? Go on long walks? Linger in coffee shops? Dive into Facebook? Would that be enough? Would that make us happy?

Happiness, as anybody who's ever listened to NPR should know, comes from meaningful work. The trick, I suppose, is figuring out what might be meant by *work*, and that's going to depend on who's talking. Sometimes it means hard work but almost always it means work that makes you feel like you've contributed to something, that you are needed. Necessary. Appreciated. Seen. Heard. Perhaps it's the Puritan in some of us that says we have to be productive to be happy; who knows. Is it human nature or culture that leads us to believe our worth depends on what we do, not who we are? Either way, what happens when we lose our meaningful work? What happens when we get older?

I am working math problems to keep my brain from failing.

I am writing a book about working math problems when I'm not so sure I can write a book anymore.

I don't know how the hell this happened.

(20% of 52) + 5.6

When my kids were young, I didn't have a job, but I was working on a career. The career was writing. I was a writer. Or I wanted to be a writer. I had wanted to be a writer since fourth grade when I began writing poems and an aborted novel that had something to do with a bear, a crime, and a magic tree. From the age of 9, there was never a time when I wasn't working on some writing project. Poems, essays, short stories, mainly. In college I majored in English with the vague dream of becoming a writer one day, but after graduation I needed a job.

I maybe could have gone to graduate school. I didn't, for several reasons, but one big one was math. To get in, I would have to take the GRE. Half of the GRE is math, and I knew that, and there was no freaking way. That road was washed out, the bridges burned, the maps lost. Instead, I went to work as a newspaper reporter. Of course! I had been the editor of my college newspaper so I had some experience. Also, Watergate. In 1978 there were good reasons to think being a newspaper reporter was about as glamorous a job as one could hope for. I moved to the small town of New Bern in eastern North Carolina and joined the newsroom.

Where I discovered that being a newspaper reporter was a lot of things – challenging, interesting, sometimes fun, often tedious, a tad scary – but not glamorous. At a small newspaper with only four reporters covering three counties, we covered some of everything, which included city councils, county commissions, school boards, crime, corruption, squid boats, Shakespeare productions, garden clubs, downtown development, sailing, shrimp recipes, and the Blue Angels. I was a decent enough newspaper reporter, and had I decided to make journalism my career I would have found time to get a lot better. But always there was this other thing, this hunger, this longing to tell a different kind of story.

I remember sitting in Pamlico County Commission meetings where the commissioners all were farmers or fishermen. When the topic of purchasing or fixing a truck or backhoe or bulldozer arose, we reporters knew to put down our notebooks in anticipation of at least a 20 to 30-minute discussion, more like an exercise in one-upsmanship, to prove who knew more about trucks. My colleagues hated this. I loved it. And not because I cared one bit about trucks. But I did care about the characters these people became when they got to talking about vehicles. These characters. These people. I wanted to make up stories about them.

I wrote those stories and many more in my spare time, but it wasn't until after several more years, a marriage, an assortment of jobs, and a couple of moves before I got serious about this writing business. We were in Augusta, Georgia. I'd just had my first son. While he napped, I realized I could choose between washing dishes or writing. Shall I say I got comfortable with dirty dishes?

For years I wrote with no success, if the measure of success is publication. I did build an ever-thickening file of rejections, some of them exceedingly complimentary. The thicker the file, the more I braced for the very real possibility that my dream would never come true even as I believed that I owed it to myself to try. I wasn't stupid. In the back of my mind I had a deadline. Nothing fixed or rigid -- more like I'd know it when I saw it -- but when that time came with nothing to show for all this writing, I had resolved as a sane and reasonable person to change course. Find a new dream.

That baby I had in Augusta was 10 years old when the idea for a story came to me in a hotel room in North Carolina. *Rose is dead,* I thought. I picked up my notebook and wrote down what would become the first sentence of my first novel. Then, against odds so long I could barely fathom, it got published. True, this had been my dream since I was 9 years old, but dreams, quite famously, hardly ever come true. I was 44.

I remember where I was when the phone rang, about to leave the house to pick up the kids from school. A woman's voice was on the other end of the line. I did not know her. She gave me her name, and then she said. *I love your book. I'd like the opportunity to represent you.*

Wait, what did you say?

After years on the roller coaster of submission and rejection, these were the magic words I thought I'd never hear. The book did find publisher. I was a writer. In my hands I held a book with my name on the cover, and then two years later it happened again with a second novel. That deadline I had set for myself? It never came. I wrote and wrote and wrote with no success until BAM! I had the career I'd been working toward all my life.

So I wrote another book.

And then I wrote another.
And another one after that.

9(2/9 + 20/12)

While running one morning, I felt a sudden and sharp pain in my right heel. I kept running. But the pain spread quickly to the arch of my foot until every step was excruciating. Typically I run through knee pain, hip pain, hamstring pain, but not this pain. This pain forced me to stop running and walk, and by the time I got back to the car I could barely do that. It was plantar fasciitis, and I knew it but didn't want to believe it. Mostly I was furious. It came out of nowhere with no warning and it was stupid. I did not have time for it. Plantar fasciitis meant the time-suck of going to physical therapy twice a week, but it also meant not running for months which is another kind of pain because am not a nice person when I can't run. I'm pissed off and barely civil.

Which is not to say I'm proud of it. It may be true that more than half of why I run is for mental health but that does not give me license to turn into a child when I can't run. These days it is impossible not to be reminded of how gracelessly I handled this temporary setback in my exercise routine and wonder that my mother isn't raging around like a wounded hyena over this Alzheimer's. I would be, I think. Alzheimer's is not temporary. Alzheimer's is more than a setback. But Alzheimer's also doesn't hurt. And if you aren't the one experiencing symptoms of your own disease, would you even know to rage?

Never once has my mother confided to me any sense of anger or even sadness over what's happening to her. In the beginning she did occasionally question my dad. Was she repeating herself? And how noticeable was it, really. Her questions indicated a measure of clarity seeping in, an acknowledgement. Maybe it's true, something's not quite right? But when every once in a while she cried, it was not over her own loss. It was his. It made her sad to think about what's in store for my dad. She did not want to leave him. She did not want him to be left.

All of this I know only because he told me. I never saw her cry, although it broke my heart to imagine the two of them staring at what the future might bring. But in a perverse way I was glad to hear she could still cry. Sadness sounded like a normal reaction to this disease. How could a functioning brain not be at least a little bit upset at its own decline? The alternative was for her to lose herself so completely that she would not be a part of her own grief. I was silently grateful there was still enough of her to feel sad.

But those tears, those moments of clarity were rare and, over the subsequent months and years, got rarer until they stopped. When I'm around, my mother does not appear upset. She does nothing to indicate that she's feeling sorry for herself or that life is not fair, and I don't think she's putting on a good face for my benefit. Her initial feisty reaction to the diagnosis --*what are you going to do about it* -- has mellowed. Everything has mellowed. What I'm seeing these days is a mellow version of my mother that I have never seen before. It's almost like she forgets to be angry, and I'm talking about a woman who used wake up every morning with a list.

And she has forgotten pain. Miraculously. For years, and I mean for longer than I can remember, my mother suffered from a rotating sequence of chronic pain. Back pain, knee pain, headaches, stomach-aches. All gone now. The most dramatic was pain associated with bladder spasms caused by interstitial cystitis, a disease my mother controlled for decades by avoiding spicy foods and alcohol. Now it's gone. Now she does not remember she has it. Spicy foods? No problem. A shot of vodka before dinner? Please.

As miracles go, this one appears to be common. According to gerontologist Dr. Lindquist, it's not unusual for Alzheimer's patients to forget to exhibit symptoms of diseases they've suffered from for years. She's seen it all: people who used to be short of breath –not anymore. People who used to complain of chronic runny noses –not anymore. "It's kind of fun to watch," she told me. Memory loss can reduce anxiety.

"People with severe memory loss," she explained, "I've seen how things that used to bother them are not there anymore. Like pain. There's a psychological component to a lot of our life. You don't realize how much you're held back by it, or how much it transitions into actual symptoms until the brain starts going and gets back to being like a 4-year-old when headaches didn't exist. When you've got anxiety, it can translate a lot of your stress into what we perceive as physical symptoms. But when you cut the connection, you might say, *I feel great! Life is good!*"

This is my mother? Alarmingly.

I call her on the telephone. Life is good. I go down to see her. Life is still good. We talk about the weather and she's happy about it no matter what. If it's raining, we've needed the rain. If it's hot, it's finally summer. If it's cold, it's not as cold as it's been in the past.

Nothing makes her happier than Honey, her West Highland white terrier. Also the flowers in the yard and the birds at the birdfeeder. She feels great.

"It's just one of those weird things with the brain," Dr. Lindquist said.

No shit.

Who even are we, really? What if who we think we are is not who we really are. What if who we are now is not who we're going to be later? Are we even sure we're still who we used to be? And how much of who we are depends on what's going on inside our brains? Our physical brains, the neural connections, the cells, the bumps and bundles, the plaques. It's unsettling. A couple of changes up there and the next thing you know, you have a different personality. If there's even such a thing as a personality, by which I mean a particular, recognizable and stable set of characteristics, memories, affinities, quirks. My mother is still my mother. But not exactly.

Who am I if not a writer?

Who am I if not a runner?

These are questions I'd just as soon not have to answer, even as I know things change, they're always changing, and I am not immune. Cultural pressure leads me to judge my own personal worth by what I do. What we accomplish, how much we contribute: these are measurements bloated with value judgments. "I'm busy" seems to be the most impressive thing anybody can say these days. I'm busy, so, so busy.

Translation: I'm important, I have meaningful work, I have meaning.

But my mother's days are lovely; how can I say otherwise? She sleeps late, eats breakfast, reads a little of the newspaper, plays solitaire, watches a little television, pats her dog, takes an occasional walk, sits on the sun porch, works crossword puzzles, and naps. I think about my grandmother, deflated that nobody needed her to do laundry anymore. From what I can tell, my mother is just fine with it.

(5 x 6) - 12

I took a test. This was after an online lesson on factoring with distributive properties, and I felt good about it. The concept wasn't hard the first time around, and the test was a routine review. I was not in the habit of acing tests, but flying through this one I remember feeling a buzz of excitement as I dispensed with problem after problem with ease. *How cool is this! Could I be a math whiz after all? Dare I dream of calculus?* Then I checked my answers.

And discovered that I missed 7 out of 20. Seven. Out of 20 questions, 7 wrong. Something like 35 percent wrong, which means I made a 65, or a big, fat F.

I don't have to put up with this shit.

That was my first thought. Honestly, I wanted to quit. There weren't many reasons not to. Maybe no reasons. So many other things I could be doing with my time, things I'm actually good at, things that do not make me feel at once furious and disheartened, flummoxed and humiliated and discouraged and scared. Who the hell cares if I can factor with distributive properties? Who cares if I can find the speed at which Sally rides to the store or when two stupid trains will meet? Learning to play the piano is frustrating and humbling and hard, but when you practice the piano, at least you end up with a song.

I did not quit.

I started over. Why? I don't know. I am not a focused person, I am sloppy and careless and often impatient. But I can be persistent. I call it doggedness because it feels a little rough, a little ungainly, like an image of me in the last couple of miles of a long run, hunched over, hamstrung and stride-shortened, face set in a grimace, running with a posture you ought not to run with, gutting it out. It's not pretty. But it's kind of like I can't see that I have a choice.

Forty years ago in a newspaper office in New Bern, North Carolina, I was working on what would become a three-part series of articles on pollution in the Neuse River. As one of only four reporters covering three counties, I didn't have a lot of time for investigative journalism. There were daily assignments and deadlines; anything extra had to be squeezed into spare time. But the glory of Watergate had seduced me into journalism in the first place: of course I was going to damn well investigate something! At the time, nobody could say exactly what was going on with the river; so I went after that.

After months of talking to local, state, and federal officials, E.P.A. biologists, farmers, and fishermen, I came up with a complicated picture involving multi-faceted culprits, which was not what I'd hoped for. How much more satisfying, cinematic even, to find a single villain, say, the Weyerhaeuser Paper Company. But effluence from farmland runoff was equally at fault. The Neuse River was polluted; fixing it would not be easy. Neither would be the story to explain it all. When finally I had finished the reporting, I sat down to write.

It was late at night, after hours, and I was alone in the newsroom. Working methodically, uninterrupted, I was a paragraph, maybe two, away from finishing the first 4,000-word article, when I accidently deleted it. And by *it*, I mean the whole damn thing.

Computers were new to us; we didn't even call them computers. We called them VDTs: video display terminals. Before VDTs, I'd typed my stories on an old manual typewriter on long sheets of beige-colored paper. No question, the computer was easier because of cut and paste and because you didn't have to use White-Out to correct mistakes. But this early model, at least the one I was working on that evening, did not have that feature that asks you if you want to delete after you accidently hit the delete key. No, it just deleted. Vanished into the blank screen. Two hours of work. 4,000 words. Gone. Poof.

How did I rage? I never have been at a loss for ways. No doubt this one was epic, the particulars not worth remembering. But I do remember the recognition that slowly and quietly settled over me when it became clear the raging changed nothing. Slowly and quietly I began to understand what I was supposed to do next. There was nothing else to do but start over. Doggedly.

Seven out of 20 mistakes on a math test? A big, fat F. I stared at the piece of paper covered in X's. I wadded it up and threw it away. Then I started over.

Sometimes math is hard. Sometimes math does not feel like a language. Sometimes math does not present itself as symbolic for how things work in the real world. Sometimes you can know math symbolizes real things in the world but you don't give a damn because math is so freaking hard. Sometimes working a math problem feels like I've crawled into a tunnel and then the flashlight goes out and I'm banging around in the dark, bumping into things, stubbing my toe, hitting my head, and I have to tamp down the fear that there may very well be no way I'm getting out of the tunnel.

So I get impatient. Also tired. It takes a lot out of me to do this math. As if mental energy were a substance that leaks out of my brain and leaves me half-witted, slow, fuzzy, and dim. Also angry. I find myself tearing into tiny pieces sheets of ruled paper, littered with barely legible pencil scratchings. Like clouds dissipating, the beautiful concepts I think I've learned devolve into a series of tricks I'm just supposed to *know*. But I don't know. There's something about me and tricks: I don't like them, I don't respect them, and I don't want to accept that this is math. I want math to be something else. I want to dig under the tricks and get to the why without taking the time to learn the tricks, and I want that to be easy, and I want there to be shortcuts, and I'm afraid. I'm afraid that even if I took the time I still might not be good at this.

On the other hand, what if hard is the point?

I am thinking now about Alzheimer's. I'm thinking about how not to get it.

There is an argument for making your brain work hard, like on purpose, like hard for the sake of hard. I am reminded of a lecture I once heard on William Faulkner that suggested the author intended the reader to *work* for the reward of understanding him. Hard for the *sake* of hard.

Except reading Faulkner never felt all that hard to me, certainly not as hard as this math.

According to Northeastern University's Dr. Feldman Barrett, forcing your brain to do, not just new stuff, but hard stuff, is a trait that differentiates "super-agers" from the rest of us. In her 2017 *New York Times* column, she wrote, "The paradox, especially in our culture, is that when the brain regions that need to stay thick increase in activity, you don't feel good. You feel tired, stymied, frustrated – but if you can push past the temporary unpleasantness of intense effort, the result is a more youthful brain that helps maintain a sharper memory and greater ability to pay attention."

Okay then. Maybe. Who knows. But here in my kitchen working alone and afraid, I can't help but ask: does working hard make you a super-ager? Or are super-agers just older versions of people already equipped mentally and psychologically to work hard?

So much we do not know. We do not know what causes Alzheimer's or how to prevent it. And if some smart somebody does come up with a drug or a treatment, it will be too late for my mother. Most likely too late for me. Nobody can say, really, what I should do. Nobody can tell me how much I should worry or, more importantly, convince me not to worry.

Worry is a well-traveled pathway through my brain. The ruts are deep, the soil hard packed, the exits closing fast. These days when I think about new paths I'm hoping to carve with math, I find myself wondering if it might be just as effective to get out of some of these old worry ruts. Change *their* course.

(9 x 4) - 17

In the mail is a letter from The Alzheimer's Association asking for money along with a flyer illustrating how the disease damages the brain. The flyer looks like one more piece of superfluous paper I might have tossed away without looking at, but now I take it out and set it aside to stare at later. And often. The first picture shows a healthy brain with arrows pointing to a normal cerebral cortex and hippocampus. The next picture represents a brain with mild Alzheimer's which shows some cerebral cortical shrinkage, a smaller hippocampus, and enlarged ventricles. Ventricles, I learned, are cavities filled with fluid. Holes. Evidently these cavities aren't growing so much as the surrounding brain structures are shrinking and so the enlarged ventricles simply fill the void. The third picture, showing a brain with late-stage Alzheimer's, is the scary one, calling to mind a flooded field after a dam breaks, ventricles so large they swamp out the now tiny cortex, the tinier hippocampus.

What you want to know when you look at those pictures is how to stop it. It seems as if there ought to be some helpful tips, I mean, if I needed to lose weight, I'd know what to do, but how do you keep your brain from looking like that third picture? I don't even know what my brain looks like now. Is my cortex shrinking? How big is my hippocampus?

Here's what the flier says: As Alzheimer's disease progresses, brain tissue shrinks. As the ventricles enlarge and the cells of the shrinking hippocampus degenerate, memory declines. When the disease spreads throughout the cerebral cortex, language, judgment, behavior, and bodily functions decline along with memory until death, usually 8 to 10 years after diagnosis.

This is not helpful. Where are the tips? What the hell happened to preventive medicine?

Some people have more confidence than others that we can do something about this, and I mean right now, before somebody discovers a treatment – a pill, a vaccine, a miracle – that will prevent Alzheimer's, or slow it down, or wipe it out. They recommend the following:

More sleep. Sleeping, or getting the right amount of the deepest kind of sleep, is said to allow the brain time to clean up some of the junk that may (or may not) contribute to brain decay. Sleep is supposed to be good for all kinds of reasons, and so there's probably no harm here, and I do feel better when I get enough sleep, but I should add that my mother has always been a good sleeper and now with Alzheimer's, despite conventional wisdom, she manages way more than 12 hours of uninterrupted sleep every night plus naps, so I don't know. Call me skeptical.

Less stress. Ha! But animal studies have shown that stress can physically damage neurons. Other studies suggest people who are easily stressed are 2.4 times more likely to develop Alzheimer's. So -- maybe I should meditate? Which means cramming one more thing into my day? Which is stressful enough already?

Better diet. This generally means something along the lines of the Mediterranean diet consisting of a lot of fruits and vegetables, whole grains, fish, low fat milk and not much meat or sugar, but you know. There's a diet a day that swears it will save your life. I guess I'm on board with a healthy diet full of vegetables, fruit, and whole grains. I'm thinking wine's got to be okay. Also chocolate.

Exercise. Leads to better cardiovascular health. Some people say it might slow the onset of Alzheimer's, giving you time to die of something else. I'm also on board with exercise. I would prefer to keep doing it without getting injured.

Learning new things. Math!!!!!! Exercise that brain to increase your neural reserve. In other words, build yourself more brain to work with when parts of it start to die. Okay. Clearly I'm willing to believe this one, I mean, I'm not sitting here slogging through math for the fun of it. I am counting on these math problems to bust open some neural reserve.

Socializing. Evidently, it's toxic to be alone.

It is so very tempting to seize on recommendations like these and to believe that if you follow the rules you'll be spared, but the evidence simply is not in, not yet. Nor is the evidence conclusive that medicines designed to slow the progression of the disease are any more than marginally effective.

My mother still knows how to wash dishes. She knows how to play the piano, although not anything like the way she used to. She knows all of the people in her family and where everybody lives. She knows most of her friends. She knows her way around the block. She is not putting household objects into the freezer although she does stick them into random drawers where my father can't find them.

The holes in my mother's brain where new thoughts used to live appear to be filling with songs. Old songs. Most are songs she must have heard when she was a child, songs from the 1920's and 30's and 40's. Occasionally Aretha Franklin. THIS IS THE HOUSE THAT JACK BUILT, Y'ALL. She'll still listen to Keith Jarrett and Bill Evans and Oscar Peterson when my father puts the music on, but when she's walking around the house, when she's playing solitaire at the kitchen table, when she's washing dishes, she is singing songs I've never heard before.

Where on earth have all these songs been for all these years? The woman who was my mother until she turned 83 never mentioned any of them. I LEFT MY HEART AT THE STAGE DOOR CAN-TEEN. Irving Berlin, 1943. Like fossils suddenly emerging from underneath the mud of an eroded hillside. Do our brains contain secret storage places where we keep old songs, old stories? Do they emerge only when we lose the ability to remember what we said a minute ago? Does the loss of short-term memory make room for things we used to know? My mother is time-travelling backwards.

I am tempted to believe all this will turn out okay.

We are into the fourth or fifth year of this disease depending on when you start counting. The Alzheimer's literature estimates an 8-to-10 year progression that leads eventually to a time when she won't remember who we are. At some point she won't remember how to take care of herself. It's hard to know what to think about this. People say we're in the medium stage. People say we're on a long, hard road. I want to say, not so hard and not so long. I want to say we'll be fine sticking right here in the medium stage. Because secretly I believe we are immune.

We won't lose my mother completely no matter how long she lives. She won't be like those others who don't recognize people. We're going to dodge this bullet somehow because....

Just because. I believe it. Secretly. *I believe it. I am whispering now.*
I whisper because it's magical thinking, and I know it, and I don't care. It's what I think, it's what I believe. I'm afraid I can't think in any other way.

Mary and I are walking in a park near my house. It is spring. We are walking, as we have done roughly every Sunday morning for more than 20 years, but now we are talking about math. Mary teaches math to fourth, fifth, and sixth graders at Nature's Way Montessori School and so the subject is not out of bounds for her, but it feels weird to me. Since when have I ever wanted to talk about math? When I was trying to decide whether relearning math at my age might be a good idea, Mary was the first person I asked: is it important? Is it worth it? Am I too old? Go for it, is what she told me.

On this particular morning, I tell her I've slowed myself down to go back to practicing fundamentals even though I've already ventured into lessons on basic algebraic equations. There's no need to tell her -- because she would know it already -- but it's been something like a revelation to me to discover that algebra is not a separate and distinct math "level." Algebra problems consist of numbers, and numbers include fractions, decimals, negative numbers, primes, and exponents, and so if you aren't fluent in all the ways the numbers work, then knowing how to solve for X doesn't mean much. I'm practicing fractions again, I tell her.

Mary, whose voice cannot hide how much she truly and deeply loves teaching fractions, starts talking about how cool it is to show kids how to divide something like 1/7 by 1/15. Instead of making them slog through all that arithmetic, she says, she can show them how to turn those fractions into decimals so they can use a calculator.

Wait. A calculator?

I stop walking, abruptly, and stare at her, even as she talks on. The goal -- her goal -- is to help kids understand that the answer to 1/7 divided by 1/15 – *whatever* the answer ends up being – will *necessarily* have to be less than 1. It will be a fraction of 1. The exact fraction is less important than the concept. The concept is key. The exact number does not matter, she insists. Unless, of course, you're working on a problem that will determine whether or not a rocket blows up.

My stare is a question, wordless because, frankly, I am speechless. Because the exact number does matter to me. Slogging through all that arithmetic *is* the point. Isn't it? I am practicing fractions to become fluent in fractions. I am training my mind to focus – F-O-C-U-S -- with this slog through arithmetic. I have spent a very long time secretly ashamed about losing the fraction tricks. I have viewed fractions as math problems. I have forgotten that fractions are numbers. I have forgotten that numbers are symbols. I come away from talking to Mary with an unexpected question: *what is math, anyway?*

"A student who can answer questions without understanding them is a student with an expiration date." So says Ben Orlin, a math teacher who writes a blog called *Math With Bad Drawings*. I found it one day while searching the Internet for statistics on innumeracy. It's clever and engaging and occasionally silly, but Orlin has a lot of very un-silly things to say about why and how kids fail at math.

When students are not given enough time to master the material being presented – let's say the division of fractions – they can develop what Orlin describes as a "muddled half comprehension." They understand enough to gut through lessons and tests, barely. But then they have to move on to the next lessons and tests. There's an assumption that missing pieces can be learned later, but later, Orlin says, is hard. Muddled half-comprehension is one reason some of us grow up thinking we are bad at math.

This notion of a muddled half comprehension resonates. I mean, like a gong. How better to describe the state of me in math class. To be clear, I was not a *terrible* math student. The report cards proving it are long gone, but it would not be far off to place me as B average, which means I earned a few C's but also a few A's. It also means I managed to learn quite a bit of math before walking away from it forever, but learning was not the same as absorbing. Consolidating. Remembering. I did not know that then. I do now.

Half comprehension may explain what kept me from seeing math as more than questions at the end of a textbook chapter. What kept me from understanding math as a way of seeing the world. As a way to think. What kept me from making connections. What gave me the anxious feeling that I was always just one step ahead of a widening chasm filled with all the things I did not know.

Muddled: because maybe I suspected I was fudging. Because I was scared. If a fraction of anything is going to be less than the whole of the thing, then a fraction of a fraction is going to be even smaller. Such a simple concept. Obvious. But hard to see if you are consumed by the fear that you might forget how to work the 20 problems in front of your face.

Math, of course, is both. Trees and forest. Numbers and relationships. Slog and beauty. I would like to think that this time around I might be capable of understanding both. If I work hard, if I focus, if I don't get in my own way.

I am not alone here. Finding myself in the company of three seventh graders one morning, I ask if they like math. No, they say. All three of them say no. Resoundingly. One of them, I'll call her Ellie, tells me it's because the teachers always go too fast, and the other two nod with enthusiastic affirmation. They'll learn one concept but then, too quickly, move to the next concept so that by the time they return to the first concept they've already forgotten it.

I can't believe what I am hearing, honestly.

I tell them about how teachers struggle with the tension between sitting students down in chairs and drilling them to mastery – which can be boring – and the impulse to make math fun, engaging, relevant – which might skimp on the drilling. Almost before I can finish my sentence, Ellie speaks up. "I'd rather have it be boring than hard."

Which is to say, she thinks she could have used more drilling. Which is to say that students who don't master the basics probably aren't going to end up loving math. Which is to say, I have no idea how anybody should teach math.

My mother can't drive. By drive, I don't mean the actual mechanics of it. I have no idea if she has the capacity to operate a moving vehicle with a steering wheel, accelerator, and brake. Most likely she does, but it doesn't matter because my dad won't let her drive, so she can't. The last time she drove a car ended up being a kind of test, a test my father desperately wanted her to pass because he resists taking even a speck of independence away from her. Of course he wants her to be able to drive, we all do, we all want to see her do everything she used to do, but we can't.

They drove to the grocery store, 10 minutes away from their house, and evidently she did okay, but driving home she got the car up to 60 in a 35-mile-an-hour speed zone before he told her to slow down. Going 60 in a 35-mile-an-hour speed zone is not a crime. Okay, well, it is a crime, but it's easy to do. I know the stretch of highway where she was and it's wide and straight and it seems like you ought to be able to go 55, at least, so it's irritating to have to slow down, but everybody who regularly drives it knows to keep under 35. It's a speed trap. The real problem, though, was not the speed. It was that she did not know she was driving that fast. She did not know what she was doing.

Daddy won't let me drive, she sometimes says and then, predictably, adds: *What does he think, I won't be able to find my way back home?*

It's kind of like a joke the way she says it, although, yes, getting lost is a possibility. More crucial are the myriad tiny calculations required to execute a freeway ramp, a four-way stop, a lane change, or a speed limit. A brain must make countless executive function decisions while driving that don't have anything to do with whether you can use a steering wheel to keep a car between the lines. It's a matter of focus and attention. I would not want to risk it. Neither does my dad.

Oddly, she doesn't seem to mind. There's no complaining, no arguing. She does not ask to drive, does not hunt for the keys, does not attempt to get in her car and drive away. Does that mean she knows somewhere deep inside that she really and truly can't drive? Or are there too many executive function steps between thinking she wants to drive and searching for the keys? Or does she simply forget that driving might be something she would ever want to do?

No one knew that particular drive to the grocery store and back would end up being the last time she ever drove a car. No one planned it. No one marked that trip as anything special. But it was, and that was that.

My mother can't cook. She used to be an excellent cook. She cooked everything from scratch in that period of time between when there wasn't any other way to cook and these days, when cooking from scratch has become trendy. In that period of time in the late

60's and 70's when processed foods began to take over the grocery shelves, my mother didn't even use recipes that called for cream of mushroom soup. On the other hand, both of my grandmothers embraced the short-cut philosophy of cooking, and so part of my childhood involved being witness to a cake war. My grandmothers used cake mixes. My mother would have rather died.

I have never tasted fried chicken the way my mother fried chicken when I was a little girl. And biscuits. And grits. And then when people stopped eating such heavy meals, she learned to cook arctic char and quinoa. What she cooked changed over the years but not her insistence on simplicity and quality. Now it's my dad who's cooking. He cooks from scratch exactly the way she would have done, although he is more inventive and always looking for new things to try. For Christmas I often give him a new cookbook. Some nights he calls me on the phone just to tell me about a dinner he made from a new recipe. He tries hard to include my mother in the preparations for dinner. He will bring her into the kitchen, tell her what's for dinner, give her a choice: does she want to help make the salad or cook the asparagus?

She chooses the salad.

And maybe she'll get the lettuce out of the refrigerator. Maybe the tomatoes and peppers. But soon she will wander away to play solitaire at the kitchen table and my father will quietly finish making the salad. When I say my mother can't cook, this is what I mean. She appears unable to see a task through from the beginning to the end. No one can remember the last time my mother made dinner.

My mother can't read a book. Rather, I should say she can read books that are funny and short, like James Thurber. She loves James Thurber. But no more novels. This is a loss that breaks my heart because my mother always kept up with the latest books and often read more than I did. We talked about the books, about plot pacing and character development, about themes and symbolism, about beautiful sentences. It was not at all unusual for her to call me on the phone just to read me a beautiful sentence. *Listen to this*, she would say. Now she cannot seem to follow a plot.

Movie plots are also hard to follow, and that is another heart-breaker because my mother had a life-long love affair with movies. Before video tapes and DVDs allowed us watch at home, she went to the movies all the time, sometimes by herself, and she would drag my father to Atlanta or New York just to see a movie she'd read about that had no hope of making it to a Chattanooga theater. If there were subtitles, all the better. A new puppy curtailed her habit of going to the movies, still, it was nothing for her to blow an afternoon on a movie channel or a Netflix DVD. She could spend almost an entire day in front of the television, switching from the news, to a movie, to an old episode of Law and Order. In fact, it used to worry my dad and me how much TV she watched. Was that an early clue that something was going on? A hint that more changes were to come? Now it's worrisome that she can't follow the plots.

She once asked me why she doesn't go to the movies anymore. She seemed to remember it's something she used to do, but does not do anymore. I asked her why she thinks that is. "Old age, I guess," she said.

I am a planner. I like to know how things are going to go. And I like to have some say-so in how they're going to go. I like answers. I want solutions. I long to fix even what I know I can't fix. It's only recently, and reluctantly, and fitfully, that I'm forcing myself to sit on my hands because it's pretty damn irritating, evidently, to be around a compulsive fixer. One thing we do know about Alzheimer's -- we don't know what's going to happen. We don't know how it's going to end, how long it's going to take, or what's going to happen between now and then. We have questions and no answers. We are learning to live without the answers.

I should maybe try to get better at that.

One recent afternoon I found myself watching a tree out my window for a long time. I was sick with a summer cold and lying down on the couch in my living room, watching the tree but not really watching it because I was thinking of a thousand other things. Gradually I began to attend to the tree and to see it more clearly and its leaves blowing in the wind. The leaves did not move all at once. Scatterings of them would move, first here and then there, like some randomly calibrated mobile, a magical whirly-gig, and slowly I began to understand that I was seeing, not the leaves, but the wind. I was watching how the wind moved by its effect on the leaves. And I began to think about the time my mother spends looking out her windows at the trees, and I wondered if she would have noticed the leaves before I did, and I wondered if she would have known it was the wind. And I am not so sure it's such a bad way to pass an afternoon.

My mother still can put clothes in the washing machine and dryer and take them out again. She can set a table. She can walk out to the mailbox and get the mail. She can dress herself and take her own shower. She can brush her teeth. She can take the dog for a walk. She can carry on a conversation when she and my dad meet friends for dinner. From time to time she'll say something inappropriate. She still flirts with waiters.

100 − (39 x 2)

When Sylvia was in fourth grade, she and her classmates moved toy cars on a racetrack as far as they learned the multiplication facts from the 1's up to the 12's. The more facts memorized, the further they got to move their cars. Sylvia had a blue car. She got it to the 5's, then stopped. It's not that she didn't want to learn any more math, she told me. She just liked the way her blue car looked on the five spot. Her mother begged, her teacher begged, but Sylvia stayed stubbornly stuck on the 5's. She knew what she liked. A clear case of aesthetics beating math.

It's a funny thing about math, the stories people tell. Most people, if you ask them what they remember about history class, or science, or English, you're not likely to get a particularly dramatic reaction (with the possible exception from people of a certain age who remember diagramming sentences on a blackboard). None of the guttural groaning, eye rolling, chest clutching you get from the math haters. Then neither do you get the gleeful recollections of math lovers. PUZZLES!

Tons of people told me they managed to get straight-A's all through school without actually understanding math. They tell me this with some degree of wonder and nervousness, as if – they got away with it! As my daughter-in-law Alex once told me, "I was smart enough to get the gist of it even though I didn't really know what I was doing. I could do it by rote, but I couldn't do it by heart."

As a country, we are not a math-loving bunch. Stop ten people on a street and ask them if they like math. Nine will say, no, according to one study. These sad numbers appear to be driving several math educators to want to fix it. One of them is Dan Finkel, founder of *Math For Love*, an online math curriculum resource. Finkel argues that math is *not* memorizing steps to solve a problem to get a right answer so you can get an A. Math should start with questions. When students are allowed to ask questions and then given time to find the answers – to work, to try, to fail, and try again, to imagine, to test, to struggle, to compare notes, to argue, to defend – what are they doing? Thinking. They are learning to think while they learn some math, and that, says Finkel, is the point.

Can 2 + 2 = 12?

Turns out, the answer is not no if you turn a number line into a number circle.

A number circle?

Let's back up.

Finkel is one of many educators insisting that we change how we teach math, not just to turn out students who can work a two-trains problem on a standardized test, but to develop citizens who are not afraid to think. People with some mental flexibility. For all that, math requires time. Time to get stuck and then unstuck. A by-product of a student given time to get stuck and then unstuck is confidence. Math, therefore, requires time and confidence.

From what I can tell, most of our teachers, no matter how good they are, are not given enough time. If you put a good teacher in a system that cares only about right answers, is it not inevitable that some will cease to care whether the students understand?

Which is bigger: 8 x X or 6 x X?
You want to say 8, right?
What if X is 0?

At a writer's conference in a small town near Asheville, North Carolina, a fellow author came up to me with a question. I knew him, or at least I knew who he was, and I'd read at least one of his books and thought of him as one of the "real writers," meaning his prose was professional and a pleasure to read and that he had something to say. In other words, he was not one of the self-promoters who aggressively shielded their prose from even a whiff of editing. It took energy to talk to those people, but not to this man, who, besides being a good writer, seemed to be a kind and decent person.

He told me that, since his last book was published several years earlier, he had been unable to get anything else published. Not one thing. He'd lost his publisher and now, unthinkably, his agent. He was an orphan writer. It was a horrible story. It was a story I'd heard before from other writers at other conferences who recounted the experience of having a couple of books published along with the requisite book tours and praise and promises of a promising career, only to be dropped like last year's phone book. Was he looking for advice? Commiseration? Help?

I wanted to help. I gave him the name of my agent and the phone number. Maybe that would help, you never know.

But he sort of did know. He was genuinely appreciative and thanked me for trying but it was easy to see he was not optimistic, that he'd been given names and phone numbers for some time now but nothing every came of it. What I think he was really asking was why. *Why?* I did not know why. What I did know, what I believed, was that such a thing would never happen to me.

The reason was simple: there was a difference between this man and me. I believed it. I knew it deeply the way you know things like the plane you're on is not going to crash. It could crash, but it probably won't. Chances are good. You can worry about it if you want, but you're probably going to be okay. What made us different I could not say, just that there was a difference. I'd managed to get two novels published and both were doing pretty well. The way it worked, rather, the way I assumed it worked, was something like this: *your first books are decent but you get better over time as you grow in your craft and your audience grows with you.* Under that system, I was right on track, maybe even ahead. The publisher liked me! My agent liked me! I was in a current being swept downstream. I was in the pipeline. I was in the room, on the inside, in the middle of a proven writing career limited only by my own talent and work ethic. I felt sympathy for the man who could not get published, but I was not like him.

Actually, I did have a bit of advice for this man besides the name and number of my agent, but I did not have the heart to give it. It came from words I'd heard many years earlier when I was still an orphan writer, or barely even that. When I was an insecure young woman who yearned to be a writer but had no idea what to do about it. This happened during one of the first Southern Writer's Conferences held every other year in Chattanooga. Back then the conference was sponsored in part by an organization called Allied Arts, and my mother was on some committee or another associated with it, and in that capacity she ended up hosting a reception at our home for some of the writers and volunteers. It was there, in the living room where I spent my youth dreaming of being a writer, where my mother dragged the extremely reluctant me across a room to talk to Louis Rubin, founder of Algonquin Books. *This is my daughter who wants to be a writer, do you have any advice for her?*

He barely looked up.

Keep writing, he said.

It's the worst sort of advice anybody can possibly ever get and yet it is the only advice that is true. But I could not say that to this good and talented man who could not get published. I suspected he was all too familiar with those words, and they were hollow.

How long ago that was! I'm having a hard time remembering even when that conversation took place. I want to say it was some-time around 2005 or 2006. It could have even been 2007, but I know it was before 2008 when I tried and failed to get my third novel published.

If I wanted to, I could go back through my emails and count how many rejections it received, but I don't want to. Not getting published doesn't happen all at once. For me, there was the initial spate of several months when rejections from the first round of publishers came back slowly, all saying words that pretty much followed the same theme. *Love this book; it's not for us; best of luck!* Each subsequent rejection became increasingly gut-punching. Also destabilizing because around about the seventh or eighth or ninth time you hear the same line, you start to suspect it doesn't mean anything.

And yet. Since when have I ever been confident of a final draft? Since never. So by the time the last rejection rolled in, I was eager to put my book through a drastic re-write. Extraneous scenes: cut. Awkward transitions: revised. Weak characters: fleshed out. Tangents: reigned in. Now it was ready for round two.

Which took even longer than the first round, although that holding period was oddly comforting since for a good long time I was able to look at the growing stack of rejections and tell myself there were still people out there who had not yet weighed in. Hope is a cruel-hearted son-of-a-bitch.

I do remember where I was when the last one came in. On a beach, at a reunion with a group of my old high school friends. My phone rang, it was my agent on the line. I walked to the end of the boardwalk where I could be alone. I was looking out at the ocean when he told me the gig was up. No one was going to publish my third book. But he assured me I was a good writer and he said – and I remember exactly what he said – don't give up.

And I said, okay.

Book four never had a chance. It was a piece of speculative fiction that, weirdly, presaged our current climate of states-rights mayhem bolstered by a Supreme Court willing to throw too many important questions back to regressive states like mine. At the time I believed in it with all my heart, but -- and I mean this sincerely – I don't think I had the chops to pull it off. Might I have figured it out if I had waited? Maybe. Maybe not.

The next book might never have been written because, before I could get it started, my husband was diagnosed with a neck cancer that threw us into nearly a year of panic and chaos. He's fine now. He survived the cancer and, given the type of cancer, it was probable he was always going to be fine once the horror of the treatment ended, but we didn't know that then.

In my bones I remember the feeling when we first heard the word, cancer. The moment when routines we took for granted and every single plan we'd made got upended and then replaced by doctor's appointments and tests and waiting and pain and heart-stopping dread. It felt like riding on a train. You're riding on a train and everything's rolling along the way it's supposed to be, when all of a sudden you're thrown out the window, and now you're hang-ing on, looking in at all the people in the train car rolling along like everything is normal, but they can't see that you're on the other side of the window, hanging on in terror, and they can't imagine what it might be like outside the train, and you can't tell them, and you can't get back on the train. How on earth could I write, hanging on so tight. I could barely write my name.

And then, when it was over?

The time between the diagnosis and the recovery was almost a year, but the aftershock lasted much longer. Eventually Bruce got strong enough to go back to work, but he had an office to go back to, patients to see, expectations, demands, a schedule, and he slid back into his old life. Not me. I was unmoored. After months of being a nurse and caretaker, I didn't know what to do with myself. Quietly I had begun to doubt, seriously, whether the world needed one more silly novel from a mid-list writer like me.

When you've stared at death, it's hard to get excited about character development and the arc of a plot. Death, cancer, illness, vulnerability. I did understand, on an intellectual level, that these are things that happen in a life that a writer should want to write about, but they had the opposite effect on me. In my heart, I felt deeply the inadequacy of words. I believed strongly that with nothing important to say, I should not speak at all. I felt, honestly, speechless.

And I was determined to stay that way. But over time and against my will, another speechless woman began forming in my imagination, and after quite a bit of time trying to ignore her, I realized that if I did not give her voice, no one would. Slowly, carrying a staggering load of self-doubt on my shoulders, I began to write her story.

I remember where I was this time, too, when I heard from my agent. Sitting at my desk in my kitchen, alone on an August afternoon. This time there was no phone call, just an email. He was apologetic and kind – he was always exceedingly good to me, for which I will always be grateful -- but he made himself clear that it had been great working with me.

Had been. I looked around and realized I'd been fired. Exactly when it happened, I could not say, only that more than a decade had passed without a speck of success in this, my chosen career. Can that even be called a career? Years of writing with nothing to show for it. Imagine dressing up every morning and driving to an office where you work diligently, never guessing that someone is secretly throwing all your work away. Then one day the secret is revealed. And you are left with the realization that there is nothing to show for your time and effort. Zero. Zippo. Zilch. I might as well not have bothered.

Now what?

Did I think immediately of my friend at the conference in Asheville all those years earlier when I was so sure this would never, ever happen to me? No. But certainly many times since then. His story is now mine: two books published to some acclaim, book tours, conferences, encouragement, but that's it. Abandoned first by the publisher, then by the agent, I am unexpectedly back where I started, an orphan writer.

What is the difference between perseverance and delusion?

There's a story of the writer who refuses to give up no matter what. Rejections are like gnats: flick them away. The gritty, single-minded artist soldiers on with little regard for success as defined by other people.

There's a story of the writer who does not get the hint. Who fills notebooks and desk drawers with weathering manuscripts that are really and truly not good. That never will be good. Gritty and single-minded this artist may be, but also kind of clueless.

Then there is, of course, the comeback story, the story of a thousand movie scripts, the beater of odds, the hero of happy endings. Might I contend that comebacks require a certain measure of confidence? Is it a flaw in my character that I lost so much of mine?

Keep writing, Mr. Rubin said. *Is that really true?*

It's harder than one might think to give up the writing habit. Maybe any habit. That thing you've been doing for decades that shapes the structure of your days. No doubt, this is what happens to a great many people when they retire. So much time devoted, so much identity invested - to leave it behind, to walk away, to choose the unfamiliar and untested! I am not ready for this. I walk around feeling sea-legged, fog-brained, walloped.

To write or not to write?

And if not writing, then what?

I am too young to retire. Am I too old to change?

Of course, no one is stopping me from writing now. No one is paying me to do it, either. Does that matter? It should not matter. Certainly I would like to be paid, but even more I would like to be acknowledged. Why it should be so important to get credit for my work, I don't know. But it is.

What do you do? People ask me, and I hate it. So deeply do I dread the question, I never know what to say. Shall I say I'm a writer? Anymore I can't. It's too hard. I'd rather not answer.

My sweet, kind-hearted, supportive, well-intentioned, successfully employed friends will say, *but Cathy, you ARE a writer. Because you WRITE!*

I smile and nod and pretend to agree, but the words dissipate in front of me. I do not believe them.

2 (17-5)

And what, exactly, is even math?

The notion that it might be an exercise in solving a set of problems is alarming to my friend Carl. To him math is not just solving problems, and it's not a series of levels from arithmetic to calculus, and it's not the mastery of techniques. Carl wants me to know this. At a dinner party he winces, listening to me describing my math lessons. I understand the wincing: kind of like if I had to listen to somebody wishing Shakespeare would have written in plain English. Carl is Dr. Carl Wagner, Professor Emeritus of Mathematics and Adjunct Professor of Philosophy at the University of Tennessee, and he wants me to understand that math is so much more expansive. More like a world view than a word problem. A few weeks later, I meet him at a coffee shop so he can explain.

He starts with a question. You read in the newspaper an opinion poll indicating that your preferred candidate has a 45 percent chance of winning the next election. The poll has a margin of error of 5 percent. He asks me: do you know why? Mathematically speaking, he means. Is that 5 percent a decent guess or is there a way to calculate it?

Of course I don't know the answer. I feel lucky to know what a margin of error is. Never would it have occurred to me to wonder how it's derived. (Frankly, I was far more concerned about the dim chances of my preferred candidate.) But Carl very much wants me to understand it and he came prepared to show me.

Here's the answer: First you take the square root of the same sample size. So let's say you talk to 400 people – that's your sample size. Take the square root of that. The square root of 400 is 20.

Take the reciprocal of 20. That's 1/20.

Turn 1/20 into a decimal: 0.05.

Turn 0.05 into a percentage: 5 percent.

So for a poll of 400 people, 5 percent is the margin of error. If 45 percent of those 400 say they will vote for Candidate A, then the margin of error tells you to expect that candidate to get somewhere between 40 and 50 percent of the vote on election day.

Now Carl wants me to know that the range -- the somewhere between 40 and 50 bit -- is 95 percent accurate. I am nodding. Also sweating a little bit: do I remember how to take a square root? People who are fluent in math have no idea how hard some of us have to work to keep up with even the vocabulary. *Square root, square root,* okay. I've got it.

But I had to think about it. I want very badly to understand Carl's global sense of math and its place in the world and significance in our lives, but it's not going to be as easy as he assumes.

Oblivious to my flagging confidence, he continues. Polling human beings, he explains, is not like checking products on an assembly line. Like on a factory floor, if you randomly pull widgets off the line to check for flaws you can assume your mistake rate will fall into the precisely calculated margin of error for any given sample size. But people are ornery and getting more so. Who even answers polls anymore? Who even picks up the phone? Is it mostly older people who still have land lines? Just how random is that 400-person sample anymore? Since polling practices have not kept up with technology, changing communication trends, or the ornery factor, several political pollsters these days recommend doubling their margins of error to capture more accurate predictions. Using that model, the margin of error on our original case of 45 percent then would span from 35 to 55 percent.

Which is why you have reason to be skeptical of polls.

Which is why you should care about a poll's methodology.

Which is why math is bigger than a subject in a textbook.

Which is why math can help you become a more informed citizen.

This, I think, is what Carl wants me to understand. That a certain level of math literacy is helpful and often critical to understanding the world we live in. It also makes almost everything more interesting. By interesting, I mean Carl is practically giddy talking about this stuff. His enthusiasm is contagious and I find myself wanting to learn more.

He continues with his example: "Suppose I want a 2 ½ percent margin of error instead of 5? Do I talk to twice as many people?"

(Naturally, I would answer, yes. Wisely I say nothing.)

"No. You need *four* times as many people. You have to quadruple because of this square root business. Here's another question."

(Y'all try this at home.)

"How many people would you have to poll to get the same margin of error in California?" And for simplicity, Carl arbitrarily posits California as having 10 times the number of people as Tennessee. So ... 4,000?

No again. (Of course.) Carl clears this up: "It's the most natural thing in the world to think you'd have to poll the same *percentage* of people in each state to get an accurate poll, but that formula I gave you never mentions the population. All it mentions is sample size. The accuracy of sample depends only on sample size."

The answer is 400.

Carl admits this is counter intuitive. Then he surprises me. He tells me the one thing I need to hear not to chuck his entire message out the window. He says:

The thinking process required to come up with the right answer can and should be taught.

Stop right here. If Carl is right, this "thinking process" doesn't have to be something we're born with. We can learn how to do it. Like a foreign language, we can learn. A good teacher, Carl says, will know the importance of teaching it. "None of this comes naturally," he adds.

So there it is. Yes, sir.

None of this comes naturally.

This stuff is *counter intuitive.*

This stuff *has to be taught.* And it helps to have a good teacher.

Everything Carl tells me at the coffee shop requires a locked-in understanding of math basics. All roads seem to lead to this one true thing. Just for the one exercise in margins of error, you have to know how to find a square root, what a reciprocal is, how to turn a fraction into a decimal and then into a percentage. The adage about learning to read so you can read to learn -- it holds true in math. You've got to own those basics to get anywhere. And if those basics are not deeply embedded in your core, you're going to have a hard time enjoying the wide wonderful world that math can reveal. And some people are going to grow into adulthood remembering how to do all that, and some will need a little refresher.

How can I not wonder if my own struggle with math shunted me into a narrow, dualistic view: you were either good at it, or bad at it, there was nothing in between. In math world I was stuck in bad land without a bridge. Somehow I got it in my head that it was okay to forget where Bulgaria is, but not okay to forget square roots, and for so long -- for all my life--I put math into this special category of hell.

I'm not sure it belongs there. Math might actually be very much like music in the way you have to work at it, and keep working at it, practice and practice and build on what you know. I think what I'm saying is, math may be good for you even if you don't always understand it.

I am remembering something Mary Smith once said to me: "Education is more than learning a series of facts and tricks. It's building a citizen capable of critical thinking and confident of his or her abilities to solve problems."

Want to know what's really toxic to the brain? Isolation.

The word itself is scary: isolation, rhymes with desolation and sounds ominously hollow. I picture a room with nothing in it and no one and no way out. It's that no-way-out that gets to me, suggesting forces beyond one's control, conditions that cannot be changed. To isolate is a verb with the power to corral, to pin in, to abandon. Isolation can happen to you but it's also something you can make happen; either way it's terrible for your brain. That's the message I get, over and over, from just about everything I read about Alzheimer's these days, and I find I'm reading a lot, drawn to any mention of Alzheimer's as if the word is covered in shiny foil.

The so-called brain exercises, the learning of new languages, musical instruments, word games, puzzles, math, and physical exercise: all that stuff is terrific. Certainly none of it will hurt you and it's possible that any one of those things might postpone dementia or reduce its severity. But the best thing you can do to ward off dementia, hands-down, according to the articles and the studies and the scientists and the doctors, is avoid this isolation business. A healthy brain needs you to talk to people, work with people, play with people, socialize, team up, get out of your house and into the world. Maybe talking to all these people keeps your brain sharp? Maybe it staves off depression, stifles anxiety, breaks up the fog that clogs a brain with self-absorption.

I think about this a lot, about the health benefits of an active social life. I read about it and think about it and wonder. These math problems: they are no-kidding exercising my brain, but I'm doing it alone. I'm writing this book alone. Practicing the piano, lifting weights, swimming laps, cooking, cleaning my house: alone, alone, alone, alone, alone. I wish I could remember to mediate, but if I did, I'd be doing that alone, too. It's only from the good luck of a willing running partner that I hardly ever run alone. But I would. If I had to describe a perfect day, my activities would leave almost no time for other people. My perfect day is one spent in isolation. I like to be alone. Does that mean my perfect day is bad for my brain?

I do have a social life. It's healthy enough, I guess. I have no idea if anybody would call it active. Dinner with friends, or lunch, or coffee. Concerts. Plays. Visits to my local bookstore and farmer's market. I have served on the board of a Planned Parenthood affiliate. I am an activist for liberal causes, and so there have been meetings and rallies and canvasses and phone banks. (All this before we got hit with a freaking global pandemic. Need I catalogue that world of hurt? I will say, I coped, and leave it there.) What I do not have are co-workers. Fellow club members. A congregation. There does not exist in my life a natural, regular gathering place that I can depend on, and that means my social world is constructed entirely by me. I could quit it tomorrow, all of it, if I wanted.

But I don't. I hope I never do. Surly I don't want to wake up at 80 asking, *where are all the people?* But what if a social life is like a muscle you have to exercise to keep in shape? And what if you don't notice when it begins to shrink?

My mother's world is shrinking. If not for my father, she might spend her every day moving from the couch in the bedroom, to the couch on the porch, to the kitchen table to play solitaire. My father – for his sake as well as hers -- is determined to create and maintain a social life for them, which mostly ends up being dinner out with friends two or three times a week, but he'll also host dinner parties. Even through this isolating pandemic, he managed to gather with a small bubble of friends. They never were entirely isolated.

They used to travel. Throughout the United States and Europe and twice to Africa. New York was a favorite. They spent several years going on scuba diving trips to various islands in the Caribbean. Before her memory began to slip my mother would talk about wanting to visit London again, but that will not happen. My father always wanted to go to Antarctica, but that probably won't happen, either. They have run out of time. Although it must be said, they had a good run. Better than most.

To get a picture of how much my mother's life has changed, step into her closet. To the left are the dresses and then the tailored suits and skirts and slacks and jackets. On the right, the shirts and blouses in silk and cotton and linen in whites and blues, pinks and peaches, greens, lavenders, reds, and blacks. Shoes are stacked in boxes nearly to the ceiling. How many times did my mother, eyes twinkling, motion me into her closet to show me the newest purchase? So many times! It was like a ritual very nearly every time I visited.

Now my mother with the beautiful clothes wears the same thing every day: black knit pants, a white shirt, and a gray sweater with holes in the sleeves. For Christmas one year I gave her a new sweater, aqua, her best color, and she will wear it if my father reminds her, but if left alone, she sticks to an old, misshapen gray sweater with holes in the left sleeve. She is not interested in trying something new. She is not interested in her closet full of clothes.

If there are ways I'm not like my mother, and there are several, this clothes thing is a big one, in spite of many attempts on her part to change me. Some of the biggest fights I ever had with her when I was a teenager took place in the dressing rooms of clothing stores where I would refuse to try on the clothes she kept bringing me. It's not that I don't like pretty clothes, but I do not like spending money on clothes, and I don't seem to have that thing she had of wanting more of them. If I already have a dress, why would I need another? My mother collected clothes, like art, price be damned, and they were beautiful, and she was beautiful, and here's the thing: for every single outfit, she had somewhere to go.

But in another way, she was exactly like me in that she did not have social spaces built into her life and so she had to make them. When my brother and I were little there was church, but she left that shortly after I did. Clubs did not interest her. If she'd been born when I was born, she would have had a career, I feel pretty certain about that, but she was raised to get married, which she did. She was 22.

Does she regret staying home to raise my brother and me? No. Does she regret not having a career? Yes. Both are true.

What career are we even talking about here? I think it's important to separate the answer she might have given later in her life from anything she would have thought possible in 1954. My mother is an extrovert, and conscientious, thorough, passionate, and committed. If in 1954 she could have imagined herself running a nonprofit organization, for instance, she would have excelled, but when you grow up thinking of yourself as wife/mother rather than career woman, it's hard to recognize your own gifts, much less turn them into a job. Had she done it anyway, had she built a career and made her own money and earned the respect a working life offers, would she have been happy?

I don't know. I know that for most of her life she was angry about how women were – and still are – treated, angry about missed opportunities, angry at feeling unappreciated, unrecognized, powerless. We used to talk about all of this, all of the time, both about the treatment of woman and about how she, personally, felt invisible. When she was 40, and I was 16, she took active measures to change the direction of her life by going back to college for a second degree, this time in music. I remember the whole thing as thrilling. Nobody else had a mother in college. Nobody else's mother had homework. Or a senior recital. Nobody else's mother was bringing to the dinner table discussions from her political science class about the Middle East. It was new and exciting and heady and a little bit edgy to be the girl whose mother was so brave and bold. I got a car because my mother was too busy to drive me to school anymore.

But the career that resulted from this exciting music major stuck her right back at home, in our den, where she taught piano to children who may or may not have wanted to play the piano. There were music teacher conferences to go to, but she mostly worked alone in that den. For 12 years. By the time she started teaching, I was already off to college and then on to my own brief career as a newspaper reporter, but we often talked about her work, about the children who could not find the time to practice because of soccer or dance or whatever, and the rare gifted kid. I believe she was an excellent piano teacher. But it's not an ideal career for an extrovert.

If you've been to Chattanooga, Tennessee, you may have been impressed by how pretty it is and how vibrant, with the aquarium, the museums, the public art, the Riverwalk, the restaurants and cafes that fill downtown these days, but it wasn't always like that. When I was a girl, downtown was the city center, where we got dressed up to go shopping and eat pastrami sandwiches at Shapiro's, but like so many other small downtowns, it collapsed once the malls came. For years it stayed empty and ugly and depressing. The cure was downtown revitalization.

Revitalization was made possible by the Clean Air Act, which cleaned up the thick, brown, hazy skies of Chattanooga, once named the most polluted city in America. Blue skies allowed for the formation of Chattanooga Venture, a non-profit organization started by people who decided, by golly, we can do something about this city, and my mother got on it. There were meetings. Trips to other cities engaged in revitalization. Committees formed. Money was raised. Projects were launched.

At the time I was living in Lexington, Kentucky, and as the story goes, my parents were driving home from a visit with me when they stopped in Berea. Walking around the arts community, my mother was inspired to bring something like that to Chattanooga: thus was born the idea for the Association for Visual Arts. AVA. My mother was a musician, not an artist, but she knew artists, and she and my dad had begun to collect local art. I'm guessing she may also have been looking around for a project of her own.

Turns out my mother, who had no experience in fundraising or starting a nonprofit, ended up being excellent at both. She was also good at organizing people, marketing, and communications. It was like she was born for it. She chaired the first board of directors for AVA and stayed on for more than 25 years as it grew into to a strong, healthy organization that does not need her anymore. For so many years my mother's life revolved around AVA. There's even a Landis Gallery in her honor. And while she never got paid, it was kind of like a job, a career, a mission. There were phone calls to make and letters to write and meetings to go to, and luncheons, and openings, and all with the clothes to match. Now she does not know who the executive director is. AVA would not exist without her, but she hasn't been there in years.

This is how it happens, even to the extroverts. You quit the organizations you used to belong to. You stop going to meetings. You can't follow the discussion in your book club. You can't remember what you watched on television. You can't find people to go to lunch with you. You stop going to movies. You don't read the latest books. It's hard to keep up with the news. The less you do, the less you have to talk about. The less you have to talk about, the more you don't need to talk to people. The isolation has a built-in motor to power it faster. It would take work to stop it. Even if you know it's not good for you, it's hard to stop.

And it isn't good for you, no kidding. So says Dr. Lindquist, Northwestern University gerontologist. "People who interact with other people, people who socialize more, who learn new tasks, are doing better cognitively than people who sit within their own four walls and don't interact and don't get out and don't do things," she said. "If somebody tells you they like sliced cheese, what are you going to say?"

You've got to say something, right? You can't just say nothing.

Right. But what if you can't help it?

(4 x 5) + (2 x 3)

Here's a story. Writer works for decades, churning out novels. Nobody notices, nobody cares. Rejections pile up. Then one day someone opens a forgotten manuscript and begins to read, and the writer is discovered to be an overlooked genius, and all those callus publishers who sent all those rejection slips for all those years were wrong and, boy, are they sorry.

Here's another story. Writer fundamentally misunderstands job and blows it.

It's tempting to blame my aborted career on idiots who don't know quality when they see it, and people who love me want to point the blame there. On my darkest days I just think I must suck at writing. But a clear-headed and honest appraisal must consider the fact that I didn't play the game right.

At the time, I don't remember knowing it was a game, which is not an excuse because plenty of people did. I can say I've always been a late-bloomer and slow to figure out what the heck is going on around me, but dig beneath that tired excuse and you'll find stubbornness. The feet-planted, hands on hips, no budging kind. I don't always want to know what's going on. Only recently have I begun recognizing my own complicity in my own story, to realize I might have done this to myself with choices that sabotaged my career. Looking back, I can see I could have made different choices. While it may be true that changes in the publishing world were happening fast and most of them I did not understand, it's also true that when I did understand, I did not respond accordingly. Stubbornly, I refused to play the game. That's not the game's fault.

At festivals and conferences, I met writers who could see that the line between publisher and writer was blurring. There was much bitter complaining, communal teeth-gnashing, and personal anxiety, but many writers understood they would be expected to take on more and more of the marketing and publicity for their books. Many already knew how to sell themselves, some were even hiring their own publicists. I should have paid more attention to this. I was, instead, a stubborn person responding to a changing world by standing firm.

It's easy now to see what I might have done differently. Might have, should have, could have. Didn't. Like I could have entered this crazy new world of Internet connectivity, started a blog, created an email account for readers to contact me. Perhaps tried my hand at writing book reviews or essays just to – I don't know -- keep my name out there. And when social media kicked in, maybe opened a freaking Facebook account. Maybe Twitter. Instagram? These days, as I have been informed, I would need followers. Thousands of them, as if the ticket for entry is a ready-made audience.

Who knows? I have been out of the game for a long time. Trends I was starting to see in 2004 have accelerated and veered into places

I've never been. It's like I'm so many operating systems behind, I can't get the updates anymore. It sounds obvious now that there were things I could have done to promote my career, but at the time it was not obvious. And I can't swear I would have been able, or willing, to do anything different.

Would my abandoned manuscripts have been published if I had?

Who knows? I sure don't. Those books, even I don't like them anymore. Can I say, honestly, that I'm unhappy they were never launched into the world? Not really. Because, while there may be gems inside those pages, all I can see now is their flaws. Plotlines that sputtered and sagged, characters that held back, inside jokes that only a mother could love. Drip by drip by drip. It's possible that the years of riding that roller coaster of submission and rejection made it more and more difficult for me to take myself seriously and led me to doubt the worth of my own voice. I wonder if fear rendered me hesitant, second-guessing, and choked. It's audacious to be a writer. It's not so easy to embrace audacity. I may have faltered in the audacity department.

The young woman who once was me, dreaming of becoming a writer, did not fanaticize about typing away in a room alone. No. Sitting in countless audiences listening to successful writers, she had imagined herself up on stage, reading her work to adoring crowds, as if performance was the reward for the long days of working alone, ripping up paragraphs, rewriting chapters, battling the self-doubt and humiliation a poorly written sentence can evoke. When, finally, it came my turn to stand on that stage, my time to perform, I gave my audiences everything I had wanted when I had been sitting out in those seats, but it was no reward. It was torture. Here's a secret: your insecurities and self-doubt don't leave when your book comes out. They stand at the podium with you.

The thrill of public validation turned out to feel like a sugar rush from a fist-full of jelly beans and it left me sorry and depleted. Over time I began to feel like a product. I wasn't just supposed to sell my book; I was selling me. Me!?! I struggled with the tension between needing to get my name out and guarding my privacy. And in this world of creeping commodification, where authors were supposed to be marketing themselves by tearing down the wall between writer and reader with social media sledgehammers, I was lost. I could not compete.

Or I might say, I did not want to try.

Why am I doing this? Upending assumptions. Stripping away excuses to feel sorry for myself. Questioning stories I have been telling myself about how and why I spent a decade writing books no one will read. Is it because I want to wallow in regret?

No. It's because the older I get, the less I'm believing those stories. Maybe this is a thing that happens when you get older. Unless it's just me, getting older in my own persistently second-guessing way. Regardless, it's kind of nice, like putting on a pair of wisdom glasses to improve hindsight.

Aging comes with some advantages, I suppose.

No question, it's been illuminating to look back at choices I made and see them now as honest mistakes. Maybe not even mistakes so much as a series of different choices. It's illuminating and a bit painful but also clarifying to recognize my own role in what happened. It feels closer to the truth to admit that I was not a victim of unfortunate circumstances.

$$(79 + 2)/3$$

There are 60 students in the 7th grade class. Fifteen are girls. What percent of the students in the 7th grade are girls?

Wait. Where are all the girls?

There's a thing about girls and math. Some people call it a gender gap. I don't. There's something about sticking a tidy name on a complex thing that anesthetizes it. Here's the thing: girls aren't as good as boys at math.

Them's fighting words, I know. And worth a fight, but is it true? How true? And if true, then *why*? And why *still*?

Researchers have been working on this, trying to figure out what's going on, because there does appear to be a gap, in general, at least in this country, where girls do not show as much interest in math as boys do by the time they get to high school, statistically speaking. And in general they tend not to perform as well. And yet the same studies reveal no difference in *innate* mathematical ability between girls and boys. I'm talking about lots of studies here that show, when it comes to natural-born mathematical potential, little girls and little boys are like Coke and Pepsi in a blind taste test: exactly the same.

The difference then appears to stem from cultural expectations. Girls show higher levels of math anxiety and lower levels of confidence in their math skills, even when they're doing absolutely just as well as their male classmates, according to Colleen Ganley, writing in an August 14, 2018 Scientific American article: *Are Boys Better Than Girls at Math?* Children internalize what *girls* are supposed to be like and what *boys* are supposed to be like. They get messages, sometimes consciously and sometimes not. Thousands of messages ricocheting through the air every day, even for those who manage to ignore all the pink in the girl toy aisle at Target. Stealthy expectations from the culture, from teachers, from parents, and from role models, send different signals about math to girls than to boys.

Of course, there are exceptions, there are *always* exceptions, but the statistics don't waver. And the key difference appears not to be the math. It's the confidence. Even now. Fifty-one years since Gloria Steinem rose to international prominence leading a women's movement that was supposed to banish sexism. It's kind of shocking to me, really, that even statistically speaking the gap persists. It may be shrinking, but it's not gone.

Among the studies, I was surprised to come across research that uncovered a few potential differences between genders. Slight differences, like between Coke and Pepsi, (this to appease the Coke aficionados out there, shaking their fists). Like spatial skills. There is evidence that males, in general, may have marginally better spatial skills, which may help in math. Take findings from a University of Georgia psychologist, Martha Carr, as reported by Beth Azar in her article, *Math + Culture = Gender Gap*. Among first-graders, Carr found that girls often use different strategies to do math. In her studies, boys, in general, tend to use memory to find sums and are competitively motivated to get answers fast, even if it's a wrong answer. Girls, in general, care less about speed than accuracy, and they are more likely to use manipulatives, such as counting on their fingers or a counting board. Girls also tend to hang on to that finger-counting even when they are fully capable of using cognitive strategies. Manipulatives are going to slow you down when the math problems get more difficult. In a study that followed students from second through fourth grade, Carr found that becoming fluent – by which she means faster -- at basic math is directly linked to math performance. That study found that boys were more fluent than girls.

But here is the important take-away: *deficiencies in spatial skills or fluency can easily be overcome by a good teacher.* That is the consensus. That is a true sentence. Everybody can be, and ought to be, fluent in basic math. Everybody should have access to good teachers. Again, it's not the math, it's the culture.

I remember counting on my fingers. I still do it.

Did cultural expectations have anything to do with why I wasn't good at math? I was skeptical. In terms of confidence, no question, I didn't have much, and I don't remember ever having much, even before Mrs. Atwater in third grade. Math made me nervous. But I would not have blamed my culture. Especially in high school, where girls are supposed to suffer the measurable confidence drop, I would have considered myself immune. I went to a girls school, for Pete's sake. There were no boys in my math classes. I was holding myself up to Karen Kendall, Jane Carter, and Mary Katherine Lawrence, not to some silly boy. I didn't even know many boys. I wore an E.R.A bracelet on my wrist, and I don't mean the pitching statistic. I subscribed to *Seventeen* **and** *Ms. Magazine.* Any lack of confidence in math could not have been because of boys. Math was like basketball and ballet –one more thing I wasn't good at.

Now I cannot help but ask, how deeply did I internalize the messages broadcasted to women, not just to my generation, but to my mother's and her mother's? How many jokes and pats on the ass did I put up with because I did not want to cause a scene? What might I have conceded because it's my job, always my job, to make sure everybody is feeling okay? Can I locate the times when I held myself back for reasons I did not fully understand? Reasons I might have defended because I believed, or needed to believe, they were true.

Honestly, considering how bad it could have been, I think I may have been damn lucky to have gone to that girls school.

In grew up in what I call a bridge generation. Maybe everybody thinks their generation was a bridge, but I've always thought about mine as being set between women who were not empowered and women who were. My mother grew up in a world where women like her were expected to get married and have children and become housewives and be happy about it. They weren't happy. By the time I grew up, we were told women could be anything we wanted, do anything we liked. But the culture we were breathing in was still very much male centered and male empowered, (as it is still). When you take in a toxic brew of misogyny and patriarchy, like racism, it's hard to know how it affects you. Nothing is so clear-cut, nothing is so easy. How could I not have picked up on the cues?

Some came from the way my mother was raised, not because she raised me that way – in fact, just the opposite – but because it was in our bones. I was supposed to be my full empowered self, but that full empowered Cathy contained bits and pieces from generations of women I never knew. I have been outspoken, I have led campaigns,

I have busted stereotypes, I have dedicated a large portion of my life to fighting for women and reproductive rights, and yet.

And yet, I have held back. I have deferred. I have choked. On a line, poised to step over, asking the question, *do I dare,* I have answered, no. More than once. Many times. I can't explain it. I hold two truths in one body. Maybe I didn't have to be in a classroom with boys to get the message.

That said, I can't just throw up my hands and blame gender stereotypes for my problem with math. There were lots of culprits, a mish-mash of factors, blame fingers pointing every which way. But I am willing to consider the idea that I picked up on some awfully low expectations and, consciously or unconsciously, bought in to the notion that women weren't good at math. Might I suggest, it was one more brick.

Algebra turned out to be unexpectedly satisfying. It's genuinely fun to solve simple equations, and it feels great to be able to say that, and, anyway, it's a relief to finally get beyond grammar school math. At the same time, algebra scares me. All I have to do is look at a new problem to feel a quick flutter in my heart that hints at something deep and hidden triggering fear at the sight of an equation, and inside my brain, a tiny voice: *you can't do it, you can't do it, you can't do it!*

To solve the problem, I have to calm down. Then break the problem into small steps to work one at a time until I get an answer. I mean a solution. The answer to an equation is called a solution or, technically, the value of a variable that makes an equation true. In other words, what is X? And each time I arrive at that final moment, ready to declare what X is equal to, I notice I am holding my breath.

But if I get it right – and I do, often, get the right answer – then I'm like a dog with a treat, anxious to solve another, and then another, because it is fun and mesmerizing, like diving into a math pool and not wanting to come out. *Just five more minutes!* It's hard to know if this means anything. Could be I'm getting the hang of this math. Perhaps it's the result of practicing all those fundamentals. You can't be screwing around with how to work with negative numbers when the point is to solve for X. You can't build a house with sand bricks. My bricks are firmer now, and that's saying something.

Doing math, and writing about math, is turning out to be a curious project. I remember in school, math was a chore that I resented, while writing was a challenge that I embraced. Chore versus challenge. There are distinctions I have not considered before. A math problem has one right answer and prescribed ways to get there. I don't always get the right answer, and that's frustrating, but the steps are clear. Writing, you don't know where you're going. With every word you're making it up, every damn word is a choice, every sentence, every paragraph, every new idea, and it's never over. When I get the right answer to a math problem, I move to the next problem. When I write a sentence, I have to go back and study the sentence to make sure it's true, to decide if it says what I actually mean, and then I have to look at the words to make sure they are the right words, and then I have to revise. And it's personal. Numbers are everybody's numbers but my sentences are mine alone. They come from my brain and nobody else's brain. Writing is risky.

And writing is hard because of the inherent imprecision of language. It is hard to say what you mean. Ideas that originate in the mind are not confined to language, they are infused with imagery and emotion and nuance and things not said and time travel and backstory and suspense and drama and histrionics and color and sound and smell and things I can't put my finger on that don't break down easily into words and sentences and paragraphs.

But math, my friends, is not *easier*. Math is just differently hard and for myriad reasons. In a history class on the beginnings of World War II, for instance, you're likely to be able to walk out with the ability to tell a story. You may not get all the dates right. You may mix up places or forget somebody's name, but you won't lose the fundamental story of why and how the war began. But over in math class, you can learn how to work a word problem involving two trains and you can work that problem step by step with increasing confidence and when you finish you can absolutely come up with the wrong answer. One tiny mistake can blow up the entire problem. Regardless of what you may or may not know, you are a hundred percent wrong. Burned enough times, you might not be so eager to keep trying.

Algebra was mesmerizing and meditative, consistent and fun, until it got hard. For my introduction into algebra, I was toggling between two online courses, one from The Teaching Company, the other from Khan Academy, both helpful in different ways. I got comfortable solving simple equations, doing to the right side what you do to the left, following the rules of multiplying before adding, simplifying, and checking my answers by replacing variables with solutions. Heady with newly recovered skills, in a hurry, racing through lessons and exercises and tests, I made my share of mistakes but forged ahead because I believed had this algebra thing nailed down.

Then one day I found myself mired in the difference between the point slope form: $y2 - y1/x2 - x1$, and the slope intercept form, $y = mx + b$, where m is the slope and b is the y intercept, and while I was working to understand all that, I was being told to haul out the graph paper because we were going to be graphing points on a line.

Really? Did we have to?

At dinner that night, I asked Bruce: did he remember algebra ever requiring the use of graph paper? Again with the look: *are you kidding*? Bruce may never get over what all I don't know about math. Um, he said, yes?

And then, like a flash of light, like what rock had I been under, I got it.

The lessons I'd run myself into were on linear equations.

The equations I was being asked to solve were called linear.

That was their name.

Linear means line.

Solving linear equations means exactly that: using math to describe a line. A straight line marked between points on a graph.

The line is the damn point.

And so, without meaning to, I uncovered one more hurdle between math and me. Because once again I caught myself picking at weeds with no comprehension of the massive forest surrounding me. Because even when I know better, I approach math on the micro level of figuring out the particular steps I must execute in order to solve a particular problem – never recognizing what a problem might be saying about the world and how it works. I am missing context. Math is a language, but I can't seem to speak it. Numbers are symbols, but that's just a bunch of lovely words strung together when I'm gutting through math problems, crossing my fingers that I'll remember the tricks.

Here's another story.

Writer manages to finish a novel despite harboring near crippling doubts about her ability to turn the loose ideas ranging around in her head into a coherent story with all those characters to deal with and plot lines to keep straight and words that – every single one of them -- could be other words. And then she pulls off getting it published even though she was pretty sure that would never happen. And then she does it again. Not everybody can write a novel. Or two. Not every writer can get published. These are feats worthy of some measure of pride, and the fact that she never got another book published does not have to diminish the accomplishment.

So much depends on the story you want to tell.

I had never once considered that story. People tried to tell me that story, and I would nod and smile at them, but I never believed it. The story I told was the one about failure, and I told it over and over again until I knew the words by heart. So deep in my heart lodged the story of failure that it was hard to sit down and start writing this book. Really hard. And it's not like it's been easy going ever since, either. No, there have been times I've almost quit. Many times.

Like yesterday.

Like this morning.

I wanted to quit because it's stupid to keep doing something you're so good at failing. It's stupid not to recognize the difference between perseverance and delusion.

It was an accident, finding this new story. Here I was trying to learn a little math to strengthen my brain, and I was writing about it, and I was writing about my mother, and Alzheimer's disease, and my own struggles with the implications and challenges of growing older, looking ahead at how I might want to spend my last years, looking behind at accumulated regret, and without meaning to I found myself writing about the nosedive of my career, dissecting it, choosing the actual words that would make up the sentences to describe my mistakes. Writing the story of my failure, I realized I was writing a story. This story had the power to knock me flat and leave me gasping with impotent despair, to turn ugly the secret places behind the confident mask the rest of the world assumed was me, and to overwhelm the vestiges of self-respect I still clung to, but it was a story. A true story -- or a story with some truth in it -- but still. Only a story. There are other stories.

I want to say it was an epiphany, but it wasn't like that. It was quieter. Slower. Less definitive. No trumpets, no fireworks, no brain explosions. More like dipping a toe into unfamiliar water. Like recognizing the insidious nature of the hijacked brain that tells me the world works in a certain way.

When maybe it does.

But maybe it doesn't.

Like a path to a tentative answer to the question: am I too old to change?

No. Maybe the answer is no.

3 (6 + 4)

On her way to work, Bess gets stuck in traffic and averages only 20 mph, but on the way home that night she averages 40 mph. Total driving time for that day was an hour and a half. How long did it take her to drive to work?

An airplane leaves the airport traveling an average rate of 564km/h. Thirty minutes later, a second airplane leaves the airport. It's traveling an average rate of 744km/h in the same direction. How long before the second airplane catches up with the first.

Two trains leave the station ...

What I call the two trains problems all fall into the general category of distance-rate-time problems. This turned out to be an important piece of information for me to understand. These word problems are not traps floating around willy-nilly, set to snag me, to trick me into believing I can't do math. There's a box to put them in. Put them all in that box – at least I know what I'm dealing with. At least I know how to start.

d = rt

Distance-rate-time problems can be further subdivided into three main groups.

The first group is same-direction travel. Two trains leave the same station at different times, the second traveling faster than the first, so the question will be: how long before the second train catches the first train.

The second version involves opposite-direction travel. Two trains leave at the same time from separate stations on parallel tracks heading toward each other, and the question will be figuring out when they'll meet up.

The third version is round-trip travel. This one involves only one train. It goes to some place and then turns around and comes back home, the hitch being that the going to is slower or faster than the coming back. The question will be to figure out either the speed or the time of one of those legs.

All three versions require the simple formula, d=rt to solve. That is: distance equals rate multiplied by time. Easy! Right? It seems like it should be easy. But I have been working tons of these problems, and they are not always easy. It's the sort of thing that used to make me furious. Why is something that *should be* so easy be so damn hard?

Here's why. They don't always give you the d and the r and the t. You have to figure out what the d is, or the r, or the t, before you can plug numbers into the formula. Sometimes the whole point is the figuring out, not the plugging in. But I had to quit being so furious before I could see it. I had to stop throwing obstacles in my own path. Knowing about the box was just the first step. I had to stop being afraid to look inside the box at the pieces of the problem.

It took sitting down with a chapter in an Algebra textbook to give me the time to get over being mad and the space to break down my resistance to the two trains. My friend Grier brought me the textbook. We sat on my screen porch. It was summer. The cicadas were churning. The hummingbirds were fighting. Grier was showing me her solution to a two trains word problem on a piece of scratch paper. The green and blue textbook with a picture of a roller coaster lay between us. I had not yet read the chapter on Equations and Problem Solving. I was watching Grier with her scratch paper and trying to hide my panic.

I will never get this. What is wrong with me?

And then Grier said, you have to *do* math to do math.

Wait. What was that?

Off-handedly is how she said it, like it was obvious. You have to *DO* math ... to do math.

To explain, Grier told me that after she retired from teaching calculus, she began tutoring a few kids here and there -- all kinds of math to all kinds of kids, but not a lot of calculus. Maybe the kids who make it to calculus aren't the ones who need extra help. Years went by, and Grier's calculus gears got rusty. So much so that when a calculus student would pop up, she would end up having to re-teach herself. "I'd spend two hours studying for every one hour of teaching." That's how much she forgot, she told me. It's just true: you are going to lose what you don't use.

You have to *do* math to do math.

A revelation.

I remembered, while observing a fifth-grade math class at Nature's Way Montessori School, two girls sat down to work the same problem. One, I'm calling her Sue, clearly was known for having some math skills because classmates had been coming to her for help all morning. The other, I'll call her Anne, was just as clearly lost. Procrastinating, daydreaming, distracted. The problem they had been asked to work had something to do with graphing the location of neighbors on a road.

Sue sat down, looked at the problem, drew a straight line to represent the road, and then began marking points on the line that she would use to solve the problem. It appeared instinctive to her to break the problem down into workable parts, word-by-word and sentence-by-sentence. Her lines were straight. Her points were placed in an orderly fashion.

Anne looked at the problem and begins to draw. Her line was curved. Wobbly. Her points were all over the place. Incoherent. It was a mess. It looked very much like something I would draw. She was having quite a bit of trouble solving the problem.

I asked her if she likes math.

"It's okay," she said.

I suspected she was being diplomatic to the nice lady who had dropped in to observe her math class. I asked her if there's any subject that she really and truly likes.

I like to write, she said.

Sue looked up from her work. "She writes poetry," she said. "She writes beautiful poems."

And I thought, of course she does.

And I thought, that's me, writing poems, sucking at math.

But is that true?

Since that day, I have used Sue and Anne as an analogy to justify my default identity as a girl who's not up to the challenge. A girl whose brain is not wired for math. A girl who's not brave. But what is an analogy if not a certain kind of story?

You have to *do* math to do math.

I took Grier's words with me when I sat down to study the chapter in the Algebra textbook and began to comprehended the notion that these trains problems are all of a kind. Some are tricky, on purpose, but there are only so many strategies to use. A finite number of tools to try out. I had to get familiar with the strategies, I had to work to get comfortable with them, but I didn't get mad. I did not let frustration trip me up. *Doing* the math made it possible to do the math.

Math is a practice. A mental frame. A discipline and a rhythm and a certain type of thinking. Slower. Attuned to detail. It is not out of my reach to aspire to the practice, to commit to the discipline. It is not true to simply say, I suck at math. It's a cavalier joke, thrown out on the tracks to stop the train. But it's not funny. Self-deprecation is a trick that will get you only so far.

When you feel small and stupid, it's scary to begin. It feels audacious to say out loud, I don't have to feel this way. I don't have to be stuck.

I can work any two trains problem you throw at me, pretty much. For now.

$$(4 + 1)\ (4 + 2) + 1$$

This afternoon I bought a new laptop computer. I picked one of three models, but tonight I can't sleep because I'm worried I took home the wrong one by mistake, which means I'll have to decide whether to just keep the damn thing or take it back to exchange, but as I'm lying here, not sleeping, this loop of repetitive worry begins to expand into the realization that it doesn't matter what I decide about this computer or any computer because I'm going to die, and so what difference does it make, and now I'm lying awake struggling to comprehend my own death, only I can't. It's impossible. How could there be a more stupid plan than death? How can there not be a way to get around it? Is life is nothing more than what you do to distract yourself so you don't think about death all the time?

Unless you're one of those people who does not think about death all the time. I am aware those people are out there. That doesn't mean I understand them. To me it seemed self-evident, the default way of thinking, to be aware of death like a silent train running right alongside your awareness night and day.

My friend Lindsay remembers this thing I did when we were seniors in high school. She called it remarkable: I called it normal. All I did was point out markers for the last time we would do this or that, the last chapel talk, last civilian day, the last annual board meeting. The point was, we all were going off to college, and we would change, and everything would change, and so it was important to take stock. To appreciate what was happening so we'd remember. Lindsay was amazed by this prescience, because after we had, indeed, gone off to college and changed, everything did change. That I understood this at 17 was what she found remarkable. But I was just doing the math the way I always did the math. Counting off moments, events, years – *yes, mark them! mark their passing!* -- because death was chasing us, getting closer every minute. What was subtracted was gone forever. Wasn't this evident to everyone?

Clear as day to me. I am, and always have been, a wiz at the math of subtraction.

My mother is dying. We're all dying, of course, I know that, everybody knows that, and anybody closing in on 90 is bound to have considered the possibility, but my mother also happens to have been diagnosed with a disease that can be fatal. There is the proverbial bus that might kill her first, but that does not take away the shadow of a diagnosis, nor does it not lessen the sorrow of watching the slow, inexorable diminishment of her mind. That's the twist, the strange dimension of dementia. It's hard to know what to do with this kind of subtraction. I'm losing my mother without losing my mother.

Whatever else that might mean, it's making grieving complicated. I have so far been spared the grief of losing a loved one to sudden or early death. I understand that I have been lucky. I am not complaining. But I am wondering if watching a slow death is a different beast. I want to mourn for the woman who used to be my mother, but she hasn't gone anywhere. She's still here. Or sort of here. Had she woken up one day, suddenly transformed into this new confused and clueless person -- somebody who's had a stroke, for instance, fine one minute, not fine the next -- I might have felt the shock of grief, but she has been chipped away, little by little.

I miss her, this is true. So often I can't believe this happening, and sometimes I want to snap her out of it, and this is also true, but not helpful. Occasionally I want her to hurry up already so I'll know how all this is going to end, and this is just plain awful. I would like, very much, to cry for my mother. Only I can't seem to do that, and I don't know why.

It feels a little like trying to put my finger on a spot, but the spot keeps moving like a bubble underneath the skin shifting left, right, up and down, anywhere but under my finger. *Here's the moment I lost my mother*, but no. *There it is!* But no. *It was way back there. You missed it. Too late. No tears for you.* I know what dying means. I know the difference between here and not here, but there have been so many tiny deaths along the way it's hard to know what to feel.

My mother seems eminently aware of her own death because she talks about it, and she has been talking about it, in the same way, often using the same words, since her mind began its shrinking.

When I get up there, I am going to ask him, (and by *him*, she'll mean God), *what was that all about? And he'll say, get in line, sweetie.*

And we will laugh.

Only there is no God, is there? she will continue.

No, I'll say.

Sometimes she will go on to describe a god-like a teacher who will show her, as if on a timeline spread before her eyes, exactly how life happened from the beginning to the end with explanations on the why-of-it-all along the way. Every now and then it won't be a timeline, but a library full of books on the how and the why, and she will be able to sit down and read through the rest of eternity so that she can finally know. Either way, it is as if the reward we get for dying is an explanation.

Reliably, she will end this particular train of thought by observing how messed up it is, that we have this life and then suddenly, poof, it's gone, and we'll never know why.

And I will say, I know.

I remember a particular afternoon on a beach with Bruce when, if I'd had machine to stop time I might have used it. It was a long time ago. Before marriage. Before children. We had packed up our sheet and towels, our cooler, our books, our sunscreen, we were walking toward the path through the dunes that would lead us away from the beach, when I stopped. I stood, watching the back of this man I loved so hard it hurt, and then, turning back for one more glimpse of the ocean, I was overcome with an urge to stop time. Right then. Stop it. Because never had there been, nor could there be, a day more perfect.

It was a moment I remembered on another particular day at another beach, watching my sons, ages 7 and 4, loving them so hard it hurt, and thinking: no other day could be more perfect. Remembering, and thinking, had I stopped time earlier, I would have missed this.

So I wouldn't stop it. Even if I could. The subtraction is worth it.

(24/8 x 35/5) + 11

Here in my 60's I am just now understanding that I drive people crazy. Some people I drive crazier than others. The people I drive the craziest are my kids.

By kids, I mean the grown men who are my sons and the grown women they are married to.

Here's a sentence that is true: for 60 years I assumed it to be an outward sign of love to worry about somebody.

When you tell people you're worried about them, they can miss the I love you part. They can hear, instead, the I don't trust you to take care of your shit part. They can hear the meddling where it's none of your business part. They can hear the worrying is making it worse part. They can hear a chorus of unspoken messages carried over from the inevitably awkward and sometimes painful years of growing up, mashed up with other messages out of your control or awareness, messages that mainline straight to emotions that nobody much understands.

It is a powerful thing, a painful thing, a difficult thing, to see yourself all of a sudden differently from how you might have imagined or assumed or trusted. To think about all the years of believing you're helping when you aren't. Harder still to change.

I would like to change. It is imperative that I do. It is the job of every parent of adult children to change. Because the alternative is what? A relationship with your children based on fallacy, rooted in things that no longer are true, stuck in patterns that are, at the least, frustrating and unproductive. This is the story of every mother I know: we have our children, we spend years and years taking care of them, protecting them, making sure they don't die, and then we have to let them go. Only there's no rule book for how that happens, or when that happens, and so it's messy. It's bound to be messy. And even when you understand this is the story of every mother you know, when it happens to you, it feels like you are the first mother on earth to experience it. In my heart I believe the success of my relationship with my children rests on my willingness to let them go. The heart, of course, is cranky.

It appears to be my natural impulse to worry, not only about death, but about things that have not yet happened. I have a history of defending that impulse and even have a name for it, thanks to the brilliant writer, David Rakoff, who died way too young from his cancer despite his best efforts to worry it away. The name is *defensive pessimism*. A defensive pessimist imagines worst-case scenarios and then goes through a mental process of handling them, step by step, as a way to manage anxiety. It's not straight-up pessimism, it's pessimism used as a tool. A trick. Both strategic and defensive. Picture finding a tiny hair in your bowl of soup. You can't eat the soup, you can't in fact do a goddamn thing until you fish around and fish around and finally find that pesky hair, which then must be extracted, carefully, surgically lifted out and disposed of. By disposed of, I mean identified. If you can name it, you can manage it: *Here is something I'm worried about, it hasn't happened yet, it may not happen at all, but at least I've got a place to put it where I can keep an eye on it.*

Of course, if you're the sort of person who does not worry about things that haven't happened yet, the sort of person who does not carry around anxiety, dread, and terror, the sort of person who does not think about death every single day, then you probably don't need this trick. Otherwise, it helps. Better than a pill. Just more irritating.

Naming can involve precise articulation, examining nuance and then reexamining it to make sure every angle is considered. But wait: is this not the stuff of good conversation?

Conversations with friends, I mean. Conversations with people who've never called me Mom. Hours I spend with friends on walks, at coffee shops and dinner tables, dissecting feelings and ideas and regrets, exploring, culling, re-examining. The incessant commiseration and articulation of how everybody might be feeling, the permutations of possible emotions, expressed in the most precise language available. Then repeated because even more precise language can always be found, slight shifts in gradation that uncover new angles that better articulate the situation at hand. And then, because there's really no end to precision when it comes to language, repeated again.

And what is all that except exactly what I do when I write? Always there is a stronger verb, always a more arresting sentence, a tired metaphor, one less adjective or one more, a need to tighten, room to expand, tangents to explore, tangents to cull, a never-ending re-examination of every word until I can read a sentence out loud without wincing.

I had assumed for a very long time, possibly my whole life, that I was providing a service by delving so deeply into each and every angle of what everybody in my family might be thinking or feeling. I thought I was showing love and solidarity by commiserating so whole-heartedly. I thought I was helping.

I was not helping.

Here is what I have got to learn -- what every mother of adult children must learn.

You cannot keep them alive.

The same holds true, of course, for mothers of babies and toddlers and children and teenagers, but when children are in your home, there are things you can do. Steps to take. Wall socket protectors. Seatbelts. Curfews. Mere trappings of control, but trappings are better than nothing. Once they leave, you have only to sit back and watch and, if you are lucky, not worry too much. It's harder than you think.

But it is necessary. Crucial.

If I throw a ball and hit you, who cares if I didn't mean it. You still got hit. The consequence is what matters. Worry may be love, but if it doesn't feel like love, then it's complicated. I have to quit throwing the damned balls. I want to go back and do over all those stupid times my brilliantly articulated anxiety smashed the opportunity to listen. I want to stop before I speak rather than wince once the words are out of my mouth. I want to change.

You might remember FOIL. Do you remember FOIL? Maybe if I were to give you a hint: First, Outside, Inside, Last. **F.O.I.L**

Here's all it is: a simple way to remember how to multiply two binomials.

What is a binomial? It is the sum, or the difference, between two terms. Like adding or subtracting two numbers. (A + B) or (A – B).

Easy. Except one of the numbers could be A squared. (A2). Or Ax. It's used in algebra, this F.O.I.L. business, when you're asked to multiply two binomials. Like this: (a+b) (c+d). If the letters correspond to simple integers, you don't need a trick. (1+2) (3+4) = 3 x 7 = **21.**

Using F.O.I.L., this is what it looks like:

(1+2) (3+4) =

1 x 3 + 1 x 4 + 2 x 3 + 2 x 4 =

3 + 4 + 6 + 8 =

7 + 14 = **21.**

Clearly F.O.I.L. was unnecessary in that case, but what about $(1x + 2)(3x + 4)$? You're going to need help. You're going to need F.O.I.L.

$1x(3x) + 1x(4) + 2(3x) + 2(4) =$

3 x squared $+ 4x + 6x + 8 =$

3x squared $+ 10 x + 8$.

Got it?

As with so much in math, F.O.I.L. is a concept some people will remember because it would have been one of many tools they used in math class and never forgot. For others it will emerge as one of those things they used to know and they may find it snaps back quickly. I don't remember ever knowing about F.O.I.L. Not ever. I don't remember seeing it or hearing about it or using it. I have searched my memory up and down, and it is not sitting in an obscure mental file drawer waiting to be found. But is it such a crime that I got to be 60 without knowing about F.O.I.L.?

F.O.I.L. is a useful tool, but it's not intuitive, not to me. It works. I've tried it, I've tried it all afternoon, and I am grateful and more than a little amazed when it delivers a right answer, but that is different from understanding why it works. It is possible that F.O.I.L. is intuitive to many people. Maybe you.

I'm also going to have to say this F.O.I.L. business is a tad tedious. I hesitate to admit this. Boring is a word I generally avoid, but this is the first time since starting my math project that I feel, honestly, bored, and I feel bad about it. Somehow it seems okay to be frustrated, but not bored, because frustration can be attributed to external forces. Boredom is my fault. And yet, honestly, do I care about F.O.I.L.? Do I want to know how it works?

Not really. I get up out of the chair and walk over to the refrigerator and pull out some grapes. I wash them and put them in a bowl. I take a load of clothes out of the dryer. I check the news. Waiting for me on the computer screen is another problem. There's always another problem.

Sometimes the thing that makes a person good at math is not ability so much as interest. Math can catch the imagination of some students and gets them excited and motivated, and *that* becomes a self-realizing loop of success. Another student might have a high capacity for math but gets excited about bugs instead. Or dinosaurs. Or Harry Potter. It's hard to pick out what comes first: interest or ability. It's hardly ever just one thing.

I am surprised to be bored. I'm also surprised that I don't feel flustered over this F.O.I.L business. I have, in fact, started to notice that I've stopped worrying so much about mistakes. Working algebra problems, not particularly well, should cause me to question the thinking capacity of my brain, but it's not. I'm not particularly disappointed when I wind up with a wrong answer anymore. Could it be I'm getting used to it? Inured to failure?

Or is it possible that the process of uncovering new stories to tell about my life is making me more patient with myself over math? Am I coming to terms with the idea that I'm easily distracted, un-focused, prone to careless mistakes, and that it's okay? It's not the end of the freaking world. I can work on getting more focused; it's a worthy goal, but I don't have to beat myself up over it. Nobody cares if I get good at math. Nobody's counting. And I'm trying. There's something to be said for trying. Right?

It is possible I am coming to better terms with how to think about math and me. It is possible that I will reach a point that will be good enough. There's no rule saying I have to love it.

$$(44.6 - 15.2) + 4.6$$

The world is still turning. So says Ellen, my sister-in-law, as Bruce is cleaning off the dirt and leaves and grime from the wounds on my right knee and face and arms and hands from when I tripped on a vine and fell face-first while running on the side of an unfamiliar road in Atlanta. My hand is killing me. I can't tell if it's sprained, broken, or just jammed. My neck is wrenched, my body jarred; I know I'll be hurting for days. *So stupid, so stupid, so stupid, stupid, stupid, stupid:* I say it over and over, like I can't stop saying it, the word hurled from my gut through my mouth as a substitute for screaming, as a short-cut for saying what I really mean.

What I mean is, I can't quit going back in my mind to the moment when my foot caught that damn vine. I felt it, like a thin wire had been strung across the path, but the time between when I felt it and when my face hit the ground was seconds, so fast I do not remember falling.

What I mean is, I want desperately to go back in time and run that stretch of road again, except this time I'd see the vine and step over it.

What I mean is, it could have been so much worse. Because a second is all the time it takes to make a wrong move and die. To fall into the path of a car. To fall off a cliff, off a bridge, off a building, off a boat, off a roof, down the stairs, in the shower, to get hit by a car or a truck or a bus or a train or a ball or a rock or a tree. Or a bullet. One second, or two, or three, between when you are full in your life and when you are dead. When you don't get to sit in a chair, cleaning up wounds and wishing to go back in time and run that stretch of road without tripping. When there's no going back but also no going forward. No going anywhere. That's what I mean.

Of course, Ellen is right, the world is still turning, by which she means I didn't die. Nobody died. The wounds will heal, the aches and pains will subside. But it is also true that the world will be turning when I am dead and she is dead and you are dead and everybody's dead. I don't want to be dead. That second of falling is – or should be -- a reminder to me that I am lucky. This time. What would an unlucky second feel like? I cannot imagine.

That is not true. I can imagine it. I can, and I am, and I can't stop. I am sick with imagining, but *stupid, stupid, stupid* is all I can manage to say.

My mother used to tell me that if I'd quit exercising I wouldn't keep getting injured. Look at her: she doesn't exercise, and she feels fine! Ha!

Here's a question: how many half-marathons does it take to say fuck you to 60?

I had intended the answer to be one. But there's an addictive quality to the enterprise of pushing your body past comfort. To the edge of depletion. That bone-tired achiness that settles in after a long run feels like accomplishment. It signals a secret satisfaction that you've done something you maybe shouldn't have. Something not everybody could do. It hints at a subtle obliteration of the self. Embodied negation. You can't get that sort of feeling with a simple five-mile jog. I wanted more.

So after the half-marathon in Chattanooga in October, my running partners and I started training for the one in Knoxville in April. Why not! This was going to be the new me, a half-marathoner in my 60s. Why couldn't this be who I am now? Two races a year: would that be too much? It didn't sound like too much.

The Knoxville route is famous for its long, steep climb up Noelton Road, but we had trained on it. I knew what to expect, and on race day I made it up the hill just fine. What I had not expected were the umpteen-thousand hills that came *after* Noelton! The second half of that race was a slog and a grind and I can't pretend it was fun, but then, -- you might guess the end of this story. When I crossed the finish line in Neyland Stadium I was pretty close to ecstatic. Also injured.

I don't remember when I first noticed that my hamstring wasn't working right, and I can't remember when I decided to admit that maybe this pain and weakness meant I was injured and should do something more than ignore it and keep running. It was well after the hamstring pull was joined by a searing pain in my left butt cheek and intermittent numbness down my quad. The cause may or may not have been sustained running of distances that were too long for me. The trigger may or may not have been running those hills in the Knoxville Half-Marathon.

Back to physical therapy for me. Naturally I kept running. A little therapy, more running. I sprained my ankle. More therapy until I could run again. The hamstring and accompanying SI joint problem proved to be a stubborn injury to treat, but not quite as stubborn as me. Teri, Brent and I set our sights on a half-marathon in Chicago the following May, and I was training and I was healing and I was training and I was almost pain free. Until a week before the race when I wrenched out my back again.

The physical therapists ask you to give a number for your pain. I hate that. This pain felt as if someone had plunged a knife deeply into my back: what number might that be?

For nearly a year my therapist had been trying to tell me that I am not strong enough to run. *Not strong enough!* That I've been running all these years on fumes. Running with my feet and legs instead of my hips and core. Which left me with one clear path: get stronger and start all over.

Now here it is many months later, and have been lifting weights, and I have been limiting the miles I run, and I've just come off a bad cold and a painful case of swimmer's ear, and now I've gone and tripped on a vine and bashed in my face and hand and knee, and I don't even know yet that two months later I will trip and fall again. I am tired of these bumps in the road. Is it too much to ask at my age to just be able to run?

There are books out there, far wiser than this one, that talk about how to age with grace, how to find meaning and purpose and resilience in the challenge of growing older. And I have read these books, and I have nodded in agreement with the wisdom therein, and I am not blind. I can see that things are changing all around me, every day, everything is changing. Kids grow up, they move away, my back is wrenched, my knees bashed in, we get injuries, we grow old, we get cancer, we get Alzheimer's, we fall, we fail, we have to move, adjust, fix what we can, we have to resolve to freaking live before we die. So why is it all I want to do is stand in one place screaming *stop it, stop it, stop it, stop it, stop it*!

I want to run without getting injured.
I want to age without getting weaker.
I don't want my mother to have Alzheimer's.

(5 x 8) - 5

I am sitting at the kitchen table in my parents' house when I look around and see it in a way I never have. The curtains first catch my attention. A rich beige and maroon floral pattern, once elegant and trendy, suddenly looks old and a tad worn. As does the area rug under the table, the countertops, the tile behind the sink, even the ceramic bowl that holds the apples. Am I seeing things? Or is it that I've failed to see them? Failed to see the difference between what is, and what I remember.

My parents' house is an old house, built sometime in the 1930's, with wood paneled walls and creaky floors, but I can't remember ever thinking of it as an old house. Only ever an exciting house. For me, both adventure and refuge. There was no air conditioning when we moved there in 1966, which meant everything was damp all the time, which meant our books warped, and wet towels never truly dried, and we became aware of the insidious threat of mildew. In that house, the barrier between inside and outside was not so clear, and I would find granddaddy long legs crawling around the shower. I mean often. One time I came up on one being eaten alive by a spider. There were two funky attic rooms under the roof where fairies could live. Or witches. Or me, when I wanted to be alone. Out the windows of my second-floor bedroom I could look beyond the front yard to the brow across the street and the valley below with the city lights of Chattanooga glittering at night. In that room, by myself, looking out those windows, I dreamed of becoming a writer.

The yard was a jungle overrun with wide thickets of old, gnarled rhododendron bushes, and two fetid ponds, and tall pine trees that dripped sap onto the cars and everything else. I loved it, every part of it, the creaks, the smells, the sap, the humid air. To me, it was heaven. To my parents, it was all that plus possibility, limited only by money or imagination. Under their care, that old house was transformed.

Central air came first, and then the gray house got painted yellow, but I don't remember when. I don't remember when they got the new front door, but I do remember when my father built the deck off the kitchen where, as a teenager, I spent months sleeping on a plastic raft in my sleeping bag because – I mean, how could anyone dare squander a finite life by missing a single night of starlight? Most of the true renovations happened after I moved away to college. Out came a wall between the small den and guest bedroom to make one large family room and a place for my mother's Steinway grand piano. The kitchen got a first make-over and then another. All the bathrooms got updates – no more granddaddy long legs in the shower. A back deck grew larger and then got built out into a screen porch which got turned into a sunroom. A garage was added to keep the cars away from the sap and, above it, a new master bedroom and bath. My mother got a walk -in closet. Eventually they would add an elevator.

Even between renovations, my parents took the great project of their house seriously. I would come home for a visit and find new draperies, new furniture, new rugs, new paintings on the walls. And the new fabrics were always gorgeous, the colors reflecting current trends, whatever they might be, the avocado greens and golds yielding to French blues and grays yielding to burgundies and beige. Paintings and pieces of sculpture grew ever more abstract and sophisticated. My father and I argued over the yard when he began taking out the rhododendrons, covering over the ponds, cutting down the trees. To me it was a sin to try to tame nature, a blow against the earth to cut down a tree. But overall, I understood that the changes my parents made to their house represented two people who were always willing to change, open to shaking things up, unwilling to settle, to let the dust pile up. And so their old house always looked new to me.

Until it didn't.

Things change, always and forever, even if the change is to stop changing. In every house, I suppose, there are signs of living and signs of dying.

The other day I came across a collection of small sculptures on a shelf in a bookcase in my own living room while cleaning up a bit around the house. I was cleaning up but mostly clearing out, decluttering shelves and closets and drawers that I had been neglecting for years. It's a good thing to do from time to time, this decluttering, but more and more these days when I look around the house I can't help thinking how our kids would have a freaking heart attack if Bruce and I were to die suddenly and they were forced to clean up this mess. So I was doing my part. These sculptures had been sitting on this shelf for so long I had stopped noticing them. I had stopped remembering they were there. I picked up a yellow one, triangular.

I'm calling these things sculptures. Somebody else might call them wadded up pieces of painted clay. My kids made them when they were little and objectively they look childish and slap-dash, only from a mother's perspective they were profoundly abstract. Works of art. The child sculptor would scarcely remember making them. Some teacher had placed clay in front of him and he had molded it into a couple of shapes that occurred to him in the moment, and he brought them home to his mother, who displayed them on a shelf for 25 years so that by now -- I don't know what else to call it but a shrine. A shrine to children who are children no more.

Now I am thinking about my grandsons, who are still children, and how they have given me a new insight into children. Because my grandsons live a long way away, I don't get to see them except for every few months, which makes it feel more like seeing snapshots than a continuum. *This* is a child at 2 months. *Here* he is at 4 months. *This* is the child at two years. *Here* he is at three-and-a-half. And so on. With these grandsons – no matter how intensely I love them -- I do not get to be awash in the gradual changes of the growing child, rather, I see distinctly how the two-year-old replaced the one-year-old. And then how the three-year-old replaced the two-year-old.

Replaced. I have not chosen the word lightly. It is a starker, more abrupt view than I had of my sons when the child replaced the toddler, when the teenager replaced the child, when the grown man replaced the teenager, and the mother built shrines without knowing they were shrines. This new starkly abrupt view has turned my head around. It's not that it's true. It is not, in fact, *true*. Children, of course, grow in nearly imperceptible increments, not in snapshots. The baby who was born in late July was, indeed, three months old in late October even if I, personally, never saw him at that particular moment in time. But it points to a kind of truth that is hard to see without some distance. It is this: we are, all of us, always the same person we used to be, only not quite. Never exactly quite the same. What we learn from day to day changes us. What we experience from one year to the next changes us. And we can't unknow what we know. (Unless, of course, we decide to hide in a cave of delusion.) It means, we can't go back.

Holding the piece of clay shaped like a triangle and painted yellow, I realized, with a measure of unexpected calmness, that I did not need it anymore to remember the little boy who made it. There are photographs of him at that age, but I don't even need pictures. I remember the weight of a baby on my hip, the fold of a child in my lap as we are reading, the feel of a small hand in my hand, the shared smile of a teenaged boy who can watch South Park with his mother. These things are in my bones. The shrine was for the woman who did not know she could remember the little boy without being sad that he is gone.

I did not return the sculptures to the shelf. I threw them away, just plop, right into the trash can. It felt like something had changed in my heart. These children are in their 30's now. They are the same people they were when they were six years old, but also not the same, and not the same as when they moved out of their rooms into dorm rooms and then out into their adult lives. Their wives know them now better than their father and I do. Their friends know them better too. This is just true.

And the way it should be. The 25-year-old replaced the 20-year-old. The 30-year-old replaced the 25-year-old. I get the snapshots but – and this is the thing -- I am lucky. Damn lucky. That this is true feels like something I should not have had to get this old to understand. It feels like something important to learn how to do, to take our children for who they are *right now*. And ourselves. And our friends. And our parents.

(Okay, I confess. I didn't, actually, throw them in the trash. The sculptures, I mean, the clumps of clay shapes my kids made when they were little. Some of them yes, went straight into the trash, but a few I saved out and took upstairs and placed on a dresser in my bedroom. The yellow triangle was one that made it out. I couldn't help it. Sometimes things can make perfect sense, absolutely perfect since, because they are true, but the heart's not having it.)

(5 x 6) + (2 x 3)

Now, of course, I am thinking about my mother. The changes that Alzheimer's has caused in her seem somehow more dramatic, stranger, than the change from a toddler to a teenager, because growing children always seem to be older versions of themselves. Like if I were to plot my age on my number chart there would always be a point to stand on, and that point would be connected to all the other points on the line, a life evolving, a string of memories, an individual with a unique personality moving along the line, shedding age-specific idiosyncrasies like old clothes. I might be a different person with different people in different settings at different times, a wadded up collection of contradiction, a gaggle of identities, but they're always circling what feels like the core of me, the me of me, the me when I am alone, the me I trace back to my birth. But my mother, it's more like she's fallen off her line. Not so much an older version of herself but a new version.

It's tempting to wonder if what is happening to my mother might be nothing more than the extreme end of a continuum of unstable memory. Memory can be tricky, as evidenced by my brother, who places the action of one of our family stories in an entirely different house from where it happened. This would be the dramatic and bloody afternoon when he was 3 and I was 5, and we lived in a duplex near Signal Point, where we were sword fighting with curtain rods and, yelling *on guard* while I was laughing, he managed to thrust the end of his rod into the back of the roof of my mouth. In my brother's version, we are not in that duplex, but in the house on East Brow Road where we moved when I was 10 and he was 8, only there's no planet on which I would have been 10 years old and still playing sword fight with my brother. Which makes him wrong and me right. And yet, he will not concede. The fact that my parents corroborate my version does not sway him. He insists. He is adamant. He remembers what he remembers, and I remember what I remember, and only one of us is right.

But that's a memory glitch. A lot of us have memory glitches. Glitches are not on any kind of continuum like what is happening to my mother. A broken arm is not just one version of an arm. It's broken. And my mother's brain is diseased. Something's making it not work right. Her memory is not shaky, it is being wiped out. Like the time she slipped and dislocated her toe but then could not remember why her toe hurt. Every day she asked, why does my toe hurt? Every day, several times a day, for weeks.

The forgetting is spreading but in unpredictable ways, the decline accelerating, but it's hard to know for sure, and some days are better than others. She *is* still my mother. Mostly. And yet, there are days when I have a hard time recognizing her, and there have been moments when I've wanted to jolt her into remembering who she is. But then, who is she?

A woman remembering songs she heard a child.

And why might that be any less legitimate than the woman who could argue the merits of public transportation or talk about the beauty of a Nabokov sentence?

She seems happy. "I'll be your neighbor, Mr. Rogers," she said, out of nowhere, my signal to know she was singing the Mr. Rogers song in her head. She added, "Anybody who doesn't love Mr. Rogers, I'd kill 'um."

And I said, "Oh, Mr. Rogers would love that."

And we both laughed. If you want to laugh, spend a day with my mother. She laughs all the time. We don't always know why. It's spontaneous. Something in her head is forming an architecture for her reality that seems different from the reality everybody else is in living in. She'll be sitting quietly and then, suddenly, she's laughing.

I don't know how I'll feel about all of this if my mother forgets who I am. If she loses so much of herself that her mind escapes her body and flits around in a life that does not recognize the life she's actually lived.

I keep going back. Over and over, searching for specific moments to remember before memory loss hijacked the person my mother used to be. I'm thinking now of the years right before we began to notice things. These were years when she resented my father when he left the house two or three times a week to play golf. I remember phone calls when she would tell me how angry she was. He should not play golf, she would insist. He should stay home with her. I remember trying to suggest she was being unreasonable.

Wouldn't she hate it if my father tried to restrict what she could and could not do?

So why was it okay for her to do the same to him?

The problem was, she didn't have golf or any other hobby. She had resigned from the AVA board. I can't recall that she was doing anything much outside her house other than meeting friends for lunch. I want to say she was watching a lot of television. Often she was in pain and frequently depressed and sometimes fixated on death, hers and my father's. She did not want to die. She did not want to be left alone.

I remember discussing the option of contacting a grief therapist since she seemed to be grieving, body and soul, over the inevitability of aging. She was grieving over the story of her life, missed opportunities, mistakes, regrets, unresolved hurt. She would talk to me, but I am no therapist. I tried. I'm not sure I ever really helped her, unless you count listening. I listened.

I'm remembering this grieving and this incremental giving up of activities, and this television watching, and this anger and pain, and I cannot help wondering if my mother gave up. In some fundamental way, she looked around at her life and said, I can't. I won't. Like a turtle, seeing what lay before her, thinking, *hell no*, before retreating into her shell. I know, I know, I swear I do understand, this is *not* how Alzheimer's works. A disease is a disease.

But here's the thing that gives me pause. My mother had interstitial cystitis that could be triggered by a dash of black pepper in a pot of soup – until she didn't. Until she forgot to have it. I'm not saying.

I don't know what I'm saying.

It is within a realm of believability for me to give some consideration to the idea that my mother had simply had enough. No more. She was done.

No doubt, anyone reading this is sure to say, *pshaw.*

96-59

After my mother was diagnosed with Alzheimer's disease, there was a window of time when she could not be safely left at home alone, but she was cognizant enough to resist needing a sitter. On what planet would a grown women need a babysitter?

Before then, she might be forgetful but she could cook herself a grilled cheese sandwich without anybody worrying that she'd forget to turn off the stove. She could take the dog for a walk without worrying about falling. But the disease progressed, and we got worried.

After a while, sitters were fine. A nice woman to come over and cook her grilled cheese and sit with her while she sang old songs or watched TV? No problem.

It was during that year or so after she could not be left alone, but before she could tolerate a sitter, when my father announced one evening that he had quit playing golf.

My father? Quit golf?

"I don't miss it," he told me.

I did not believe him.

My father had been playing golf since forever, since he was a young boy playing with his dad, and for part of that expanse of time he was a scratch player, meaning he was good enough to make par on every hole. It's not unreasonable to say that golf has been as much a part of his life as his career as an oral surgeon, and while he's had other hobbies -- woodworking, gardening, model trains, playing the upright bass, tennis, cooking -- golf has been a constant. Once he retired, he managed to play two or three times a week.

Too many times, if you asked my mother. Often and bitterly she complained, resenting the fact that he would leave her at home alone, although I suspected the problem was bigger than time. Golf triggered in her old and deep scars of feeling left out and unheard. And for good reason. The way it was when she was a young woman, newly married, full of life -- the men played golf, the women sat around and did ... what? Talked about flower arranging? What were they supposed to do? The question plagued my mother. The women were supposed to wait for the men to come home and tell them about their golf games. For my mother, golf grew to represent a universe of forces marshaled to diminish women.

I'm not crazy about golf either. I cringe at the money and privilege and absolutely see its glaring connection to patriarchy and white supremacy, but I'm not triggered by it. Golf means nothing to me, personally. It is not difficult for me to understand that my dad, as well as my husband, love this game for reasons unrelated to patriarchy and white supremacy, and so it's easy for me to separate their love for golf from the toxicity of *golf culture*. I would no more tell Bruce to quit golf than he would tell me to quit running, but I was never able to convince my mother that any of that was true.

These days, of course, she doesn't care. She does not appear to remember to be angry at golf or white male patriarchy. So much of who my feisty mother was revolved around that anger. Even if now she were to remember all the things that used to make her angry, she does not seem to be connected to that anger.

The irony was flabbergasting. My father quit playing after my mother stopped caring.

Now I am happy he can play again. Relieved, mostly. When you read about Alzheimer's, you learn about the caregivers, about the strain on their bodies and their minds, about how you have to take care of the caregivers. From the beginning, I have been as concerned about my father's health as my mother's. That evening when he was telling me he did not miss golf, all I heard was evidence of his self-less sense of duty kicking in. Perhaps it was a sacrifice, but sacrifice is *what one does.* Duty and responsibility guide my father's moral compass. But sacrifice can be deadly.

And so I told him. He should not quit golf! He should take care of himself! Surely there was a solution. Some sort of middle path. Some way to win/win.

My father then tried to explain. My mother's short-term memory was shot, the confusion was getting worse, but some days were better than others. His days were filled with projects, building things, planting things, interspersed with time spent with her, working crossword puzzles, watching a movie, making cookies. They went to the grocery store together. They took walks. There was a rhythm to their days, and as he was telling me about it, I realized that my father was doing exactly what he wanted to be doing. We were not talking about sacrifice or even a sense of duty. It's like when you have a baby and there's a party you could go to but you'd rather stay home. What you can't know until you are a parent is that staying home is better than the party. What you want is to be with that baby.

My dad wants to be with my mother. You can die fast or you can die slow. Both are hard for the ones left behind, but the slow death gives you time to say goodbye. My parents are spending this time saying goodbye, and my father understands that, and he wants to do it right.

This is the story of a long marriage. There are times in a long marriage that feel insane, I know, because I'm in one, too. When this person you've lived with all this time *still* doesn't completely get you. Does not listen, does not speak, does not change. Then there are all those other times when this person is the only person you want to be with now, and forever, because you fit together, because you make each other laugh, because there's always something surprising and lovely you don't yet know about each other, because even now I catch myself gasping when he walks into a room, because the well of love is always – always -- deeper than you had imagined, because it is impossible to imagine ever saying goodbye.

2 (20/2 + 9)

Everybody told me I was going to love geometry. Maybe not everybody, but a lot of bodies. *Don't you quit before you get to geometry:* I was told over and over. Geometry: *that's the fun math,* they would tell me.

But of course. What is geometry but shapes? Circles and squares and triangles. Rectangles and hexagons and cylinders and cubes. Kids' stuff! Stuff you can pick up in your hands. Tangible. Colorful. Toy-like. As a bonus, my introduction to geometry promised I would be entering a place where no faith is required. Where things don't claim to be true until after you have a chance to prove them true. In geometry, you don't simply learn that the angles of a triangle always equal 180 degrees -- you get to prove it.

Yet right away I was hit with a flood of vocabulary. Collinear, coplanar, postulates, axioms, acute angle, right angle, obtuse angle, straight angle, reflex angle, congruent angle, vertex, supplementary angles, complimentary angles, parallelogram, rhombus, and more.

Most of the terms I knew already, or could at least guess at, but the effect struck me like a ticket for entry, steeper than what was required to start algebra. Like before you can get into the room where all the fun shapes are, you have to get over this hurdle. Geometry expects you to memorize its language before you embark.

After the vocabulary came the formulas, and I had to memorize them, and this might be a good time to picture me throwing up my hands, because shouldn't you be able to solve a freaking math problem without them?

No. The answer is no.

Geometry turns out to be pretty good at demonstrating the step-by-step math that goes into devising all these formulas, and so I cannot say they don't make sense. They are not arbitrary. You could, if you wanted to, go through all those-step-by-steps on the way to solving each and every problem. Or you could memorize the formulas. I surrender. The formulas work. Believe it, use them, and move on.

$A = bh$

$A = \frac{1}{2} bh$

$A - \frac{1}{2} (b1 + b2)h$

$C = 2 \, pi \, r$

$A = pi \, r \, squared$

$V = LWH$

And so many more.

Formulas. Like commas. Tools you need to get the work done. Once I overcame the hurdle of my own stubbornness, I plunged into the happy project of calculating the measurement of angles, the length of lines, the area of circles and trapezoids, and with that came, once again, the thrill of getting a right answer. That rush of pride. That hit of relief. And once again I discovered I knew more than I'd assumed.

What is a hypotenuse?

Turns out, I knew it. If you'd asked me, I would have hesitated: *do I know what is a hypotenuse?* But on the page my eyes went directly to the side of the triangle opposite the right angle. Remembering was like a box, opening slowly. It never ceases to surprise, what all's packed inside a single brain.

But was it fun? This geometry, the fun math?

Honestly, it felt like a whole lot of puzzle solving. It kind of made me anxious, and I would not call it easy. It was sitting down and focusing and trying, first, to discover what I was being asked to solve. Then, which tool to use to solve it. Then plugging in the known numbers before gutting through the arithmetic, one step followed by another, trying to remember to check my answers along the way. Finally, coming out the other end with an answer. No question, there is the satisfaction that comes from doing something hard. But fun? Not like eating ice cream. Or reading a novel. Or talking to a friend. Or taking a walk. Or listening to music. Circles are pretty. But math is math.

I need a teacher. I had come to the same conclusion when I thought I was rocking it in Algebra, until I hit the chapter on functions and then fell apart. Total spaz out. I can manage to teach math to myself, but only so far. Basic concepts, I can say that I have mastered them, but to say more is to deceive. Solving difficult problems makes my head hurt. It's the good kind of hurt, I suppose, that comes from working hard and feeling tired, but there comes a point when it's too much. When the math gets too complicated, and I start worrying whether certain concepts are beyond my brain's capacity, and then I have to stop.

And then I have to stop to consider, it doesn't have to be my brain, necessarily. Maybe what I need is a teacher.

To master algebra to the level of a competent eighth grader, geometry to the level of an average ninth grader, I would need a teacher to work with me, and I would need homework, and I would need time. That's just the truth, and there's nothing wrong with it. There is a gulf between knowing how to read and interpreting *The Waste Land* by T.S. Elliot. For the latter, you might need a teacher. That's all I'm saying.

Here's something else that might be true. I may have gone as far with math as I need to go. I have done what I set out to do: no longer do I consider myself innumerate. Innumerate is when you don't know how shop a 40 percent off sale – not when you don't remember how to find the domain of a radical function. I have reached a point where I can decide how much more math might prove interesting to me. Maybe I will decide to go further in geometry. Or go on to trigonometry. Or learn statistics. Or maybe I will decide to learn Spanish instead. There's more than one way to shake up a brain.

15% of 60 + 3(9 + 1)

Already I feel old.

In an essay about aging, the late poet Donald Hall claimed old people are a separate form of life. He was not suggesting that old people feel different – not counting a varying list of physical aches and ailments. What he meant was, old people are perceived as separate by young people, and treated as such, and therefore made to feel old, a great deal older than they may feel inside their hearts. In my heart, I'm still 25. More or less.

By old, Hall meant older than 80 – his collection, after all, is entitled ESSAYS AFTER 80 -- but here in my 60s while I'm still relatively healthy in body and mind I have caught glimpses of what it's like to be invisible. I've not always cared for the attention of men, have not spent massive amounts of time and money on my appearance, and don't go out of my way to try to look younger; still, it hurts when no one is surprised when I inquire about the senior discount. I don't know why it should hurt, but it does.

A friend recently survived a serious health scare. He's older than I am, closing in on 80 at the time, but keeping in shape mentally and physically, and so you might be hard pressed to guess his age if you were to meet him. So it was a surprise, and very scary, for him to get sick like that and so suddenly. As I said, he survived, but it shook him deeply, and later he described a feeling of being sidelined.

Sidelined. Shoved back. Overlooked. Disregarded. Invisible.

And I was shocked to hear him say it, and I was tempted to talk him out of it. *What do you mean, sidelined? You can't be sidelined unless you let people sideline you.* It was clear, from his mouth to my ears, that he had allowed the eyes of other people, sympathetic to his condition, to shape how he felt about his age.

So screw them. That's the spirit. Don't let the sideliners sideline you.

It's the easiest thing in the world to tell somebody else not to feel old.

I cannot argue that part of aging is math. 60 + 1 is never 59. Graying hair and overused joints do not care how young the heart might be. For my own journey, what I look like does not matter as much as the fact that I'm inching toward death. Inching or lurching or leaping, depending on how long I've got. And because I can't know how long that is, I feel an increasingly desperate yearning to make the days count.

It's this, the urgency of time running out, that has me thinking about habits that persist unquestioned. Patterns that drive what I think and say and do. Entrenched, reflexive patterns such as how quick I am to give ground even when ground is not asked for. In meetings, for instance, I feel myself assuming that whatever I might have to say is not as important as the opinions of the 20 and 30 and 40-year-old women in the room. It's a story I'm telling myself—that the younger women have more power -- and it may even be true. But why am I telling myself this story?

I am aware that the young women may be telling stories of their own, thinking their opinions pale before mine since I've been around so long and, wearing my well-worn mask of authority and conviction, can articulate my point of view. Insecurity inflicts self-doubt indiscriminately.

It doesn't matter. Whether or not they can sense it, I can. There's a shift going on. They know the lingo, they feel the pulse, their sun is rising and mine is setting.

But wait. Who is calling whom old?

I am remembering a story my mother loves to tell about when she and her brother Raymond were on a playground, and one of the neighborhood boys kept stepping on Raymond's fingers as he tried to climb up the ladder to the slide. One of the older boys. A bully, my mother called him. She would have been around 7 or 8, her brother around 4 or 5. I can picture it: little Raymond following the big boy up the ladder, the big boy stopping, the big boy sneakily stepping back down onto Raymond's fingers, "accidently." My mother saw it happen. She knew it was no accident. Cut it out, she told the bully, but bullies never listen. He did it again. That was all my mother had to see. She marched straight back to her house, opened a kitchen drawer, and pulled out a knife.

"What are you going to do with that knife?" asked her grand-mother, who happened to be in the kitchen. Luckily. For the boy and my mother.

"I'm going to kill him," my mother said.

Who knows, she might have. Nobody messed with my mother. Except of course her grandmother, my great-grandmother, who gently convinced my mother to reconsider.

It's a funny story. Only for me it's complicated. Because anybody messing with me or my little brother would have had an easier time of it. I was a little more cautious, a little more timid, a little unsure, and a little less brave, and it used to drive my mother crazy. She did not understand it.

Why don't you stand up for yourself?

I don't know.

I could say, I do. Just not the same way you do.

I could say, harmony is more important than getting my way.

I could say, I never know I'm being bullied until it's over.

I could say, I'm not worth it.

I could say, I'm afraid.

I could say, I will. One of these days.

Giving ground when ground is not asked for has been a part of how I move through the world for a very long time. It could be gendered. It probably is. The result of being born in 1956 and growing up in a patriarchal culture signaling in big ways and small that giving ground is what women are supposed to do. Which explains everything about why my mother was so intent on seeing me stand up for myself. Which is why she was right.

I have been wondering if I actually ever believed I was a writer. A real writer, I mean. Even in those years when I was publishing books, traveling to bookstores, speaking at conferences; didn't it all sort of feel like I was playing a role, donning a costume, reciting lines that were not my own? An imposter, that is the trope that even the most successful writers claim to feel, which does not make it any less real for me. Writing is an audacious act. You have to believe you have something to say. And then you have to believe you have a particularly skillful way of saying it. And then you have to believe that what you have to say is worth the time and trouble for other people to read.

Listen to me.

My voice never was full-throated. I did not claim the ground I stood on. I told myself a story that being a real writer was maybe something other people did. But not me.

How do we spend our days? How do we decide what is old and if we're there yet? Are old patterns worth breaking? I got to be 60 without knowing much about math – now I'm trying to fix it. What else might I try to fix? How might I accept the right to claim the space I still take up in the world? How might I do that without feeling guilty?

On the other hand, how hard should I fight against changes that aging *will* bring whether I like it or not? Are there limits to how much I can run? Am I foolish to think it's nothing more than adding one mile, and then another? And then another. What limitations could there be besides time and will?

Age. My latest injuries forced me to concede that I can't simply run and expect my body to keep up, not anymore. If I want to run longer, I will have to get stronger. The younger version of me didn't have to think about any of that, but the 60-year-old has to. There are 80-year-olds still running marathons – good for them -- and if I were to get strong enough and flexible enough I might be able to do that too. Or not. Those people are not me, and there are joints to be considered. Tendons. Ligaments. So I'm not sure anymore. Really and truly, there may be a distance that my particular body at my particular age simply cannot run. We'll see.

Is it part of the wisdom of age to accept where the limits are? Not giving up, not giving in, but not making shit up, either. Rejecting magical thinking. Soberly analyzing the evidence for evidence of truth.

Then what about my brain? Are there limitations there, too? Is it wiser to accept them or fight like hell? What about the capacity for the brain to change? Is a 60-year-old brain capable of constructing different patterns to see the world with? I do not know.

I am not the first person to hit 60 and wonder what the hell happened. It's a thing, I think, to reach a certain age and find yourself looking back. Looking back at my life is kind of like reading *Absalom, Absalom* again for the fourth time: I'm not seeing it the same way I did the first go-round. I feel the same. But I am not the same. I am asking new questions. Like, how much time do I want to give over to worrying about things that have not yet happened? Like, how much control can I let go?

Like how long will I allow fear to diminish me?

Like, do I even want to be a writer anymore?

And if not a writer, then what?

Or is writing the keystone to my heart?

I don't yet have an answer. Not having an answer is paralyzing.

It matters what you to do with your life. What you decide to do. With the years of your life, and not just the years but the days, the hours, the minutes, from the minute you get out of bed until you go to sleep again. Paralysis feels like I'm giving my life away in swaths like hair pulled out by the fistful. How many more days will I be willing to end, saying, I did not do what I set out to do?

On the other hand, how many more days do I need to waste looking back with regret? Because I could, if I wanted to think in ways unsubscribed by my culture, say my career was raising my sons. It's not nothing to raise children. It's not nothing to write a book. In my life so far I have been a writer and a mother. It should be enough.

Now, what?

I would like to believe I'm not too old to change my life, to start a new career, to fill my days differently. I want to believe I'm not too old to change the way I move in the world. As a parent. A wife. A friend. Throughout my whole life I have been a person who has believed in my own will to exact change, and yet I find myself not knowing if will is enough anymore. Can I will myself to become less distracted? Calmer? More confident? Less afraid?

It's hard. It's also strangely fascinating, suddenly, to see myself in new ways, to question assumptions, to re-examine my view of the world. And yet. If I can't change what I do about it, it's nothing more than a mind game.

Why math?

It is a math teacher's burden to be compelled to answer this question repeatedly in one form or another.

Why do I have to learn this stuff?

What's it good for?

I'll never have to use it.

I never liked math but I would not have questioned the point of learning it. The point seems obvious -- learning things is good for you. You don't have to like it, but it won't hurt you. Why take piano lessons if you're never going to be a musician? Because it makes you think. Because it teaches patience and persistence. Because it makes your world bigger.

Why learn math? See above.

Not everybody's going to agree on this point. I'm not sure you can convince a kid who does not believe in thinking for thinking's sake to embrace the struggle. *Why do I have to do this* is not an insane question.

As a high school math teacher, Sharon Rasch gets asked versions of the question every year, several times a year, and she'll pull out real world examples as answers. If you want to buy a new car, for instance, you'll need to understand how compounding interest works if you don't want to end up paying twice as much as the car is worth over three or four years. "I want my students to have the tools to understand these things," she says.

These days, of course, students have plenty of tools. They have cell phones. How much math do they need to know if they're carrying calculators around in their pockets? Again, the question is not insane.

Why math? Here's what the math teachers told me.

Kids have no idea what they are going to do when they grow up.

No 6th grader can assume she'll never need to use math.

Kids can't decide what they like, what they don't like, what they're good at, what they want to work on, unless they are exposed to everything. There's a big, wide world of possibility: why shut it down early?

You can't reject what you don't know.

You can't love what you've never tried.

Math is not just one thing. It's arithmetic and algebra but also logic and statistics. It can bend toward engineering and physics but also toward philosophy. A kid who hates fractions might love geometry.

A kid who hates geometry might love calculus.

Big dreams may need a little math to come true. An 8th-grader who wants to work on climate change may not realize she's going to need some math.

Math is not a series of problems in a textbook. Math is training for the solving of problems, all kinds of problems, and that means ascertaining what a problem is, honing definitions, descriptions, developing strategies, breaking big tasks into small steps, communicating differing strategies. It's a map for navigating the world.

Math is not just the solving of puzzles. It is a key to unlocking the disciplined skill involved in critical thinking. If I were to say the price of eggs rose by 50 percent one day and then fell by 50 percent the next week, you might be tempted to think we were back where we started with those eggs. You would be wrong.

Math is everywhere. Kids may not think they'll need it when they grow up, but they will. Unless they figure out how to work around it, hiding what they don't know, feeling stupid, kicking themselves for not learning more math when they had the chance.

Math is more than a subject in school. That's the message I got from every teacher I talked to. It's a fine thing to know how to work with fractions but it's not enough. There appears to be a difference between doing math and understanding it. Maybe I should have known that, but then I never took the time to think about math in any clear way. Math was a jumble of concepts and procedures I could not make sense of, and so I did not try.

That's not fair to math.

30% of 96 + 12..2

There's a photograph of me sitting on the floor in front of the fireplace in the den of the house on Woodbine Way where we lived when I was roughly between the ages of 6 and 10. I'm probably around 8 in this picture. Sitting on the floor to my left is my brother, two years younger, and in a chair to my right is my mother. I'm assuming my dad is the one who took the picture. It's Christmastime and we are stringing popcorn. There's a bowl full on the floor between my brother and me. I am holding string.

Stringing popcorn was not something we did in our family. I don't remember another Christmas before or since when stringing popcorn seemed like a good idea, for good reason. Stringing popcorn is harder than it looks and not worth it, but you would not know that looking at the photograph. In the photograph, we all look happy, although if you know what to look for, my smile is tinged with the desperation of trying awfully hard to look happier than I feel. This is what I remember. I was being silly. I suspect I'd crossed some line into more than silly. It was Christmas. We were sticking needles into popcorn kernels, for Christ's sake.

Across that line my voice had grown loud, too loud, and maybe shrill or shrieky or giggly or boisterous or irritating. It's possible I'd stopped making sense. On purpose. Because I was being silly. It's possible I had gotten out of hand, and so at some point my mother snapped at me. *Stop it. Cut it out. Calm down.* I don't remember the words she used. The words don't matter. What mattered was what she meant, or more to the point, *what I understood her to mean,* which is not necessarily the same thing. In my mind what happened is that at home, surrounded by people I loved, free to be my true self, which at that moment meant unconstrained and uninhibited, my mother told me to stop it and, instantly, I felt ugly. Exposed, inappropriate, out of control, embarrassed, and ashamed. It was as if the one person in the world who saw me for who I really was had just told me that something was wrong with me.

I doubt my mother remembers that evening. And what I mean is, the mother who was my mother when her memory was still intact. She would not have remembered it because nothing about it was memorable except for maybe the stringing of the popcorn part. But not the snapping at me part, and I am certain she did not mean her words to strike me with such force. She was not making any sort of judgment on my character. I suspect she was tired and I was getting on her nerves.

Listen, I'm a mother, a grandmother, and a relatively sane, functioning adult, and kids – all kids, any kid -- can get on your nerves. It's hard not to snap. And it is, in fact, the job of a parent to teach children what the rules are, how to behave, how to be in the world with respect and self-control. Certainly I tried to be that kind of parent. And I can't help but wonder if I ever said anything to my sons that cut them so deeply. Some offhand remark born from a random impatient or distracted moment. I desperately hope not, but probably. I can't guarantee there's no memory of words I have long forgotten that wounds them still. Don't we all have the capacity to hurt people we love even when we don't mean to? Especially when we don't mean to.

The question I am asking now that I've turned 60 is this: why did that eight-year-old girl so quickly embody ugliness and shame?

It was easy to forgive my mother for that evening. If there were a way to count the times she snapped at me, that number would be swamped by the times she was my champion, my biggest fan, my ardent believer, my best listener, my comrade in arms. The more relevant question is, have I forgiven myself for getting out of hand? I don't know. I don't think so. She was not yet brave, that little girl, and I don't think I've forgiven her for that, either.

For the crime of getting out of hand, what should the penalty be?

I worry that I am sometimes considered a sort of emotional hysteric by people who know me, friends and members of my family. I don't think it's always true or fair, and I can point to times when I have been the rock: when somebody's sick, or needs to get somewhere, or find something that's lost, but those times don't seem to counter the impression that I over-worry, overreact, overthink. I can try to defend myself. I can explain that what looks like overreacting is only me steeling myself by talking things out, employing defensive pessimism as a coping tool. Nobody seems convinced.

They have no idea what I don't say. All the words I choke back. All the opinions I keep to myself. All the worry I sequester.

Still. I have been wondering. Is my overreacting, overthinking, and over-worrying really necessary? Could my defense be rationalization? Do my emotions tend further toward hysteria than is called for? Might it be prudent to pay attention to what my friends and family are picking up on? To the space I take up in the world? To the possibility that I could be wrong?

Is this what happens when you turn 60? Do you have a birthday and then, along with presents, you open an inquiry into everything you think you believe? Your thoughts, your choices, your career, your behavior, your emotional state, your assumptions, your life? Do you lay open the possibility that you may have been mistaken, that your point of view was not necessarily reliable, after all? Do you consider the options for change? Do you fear it's too late?

I could stand to worry less. I could get a grip on what I can and can't control. I could resist the temptation to over share. I could work on not jumping all the guns.

On the other hand, a part of who I am when I am passionately histrionic and hyperbolic could be the me of me. If this is my core, how much changing can I reasonably expect?

The photograph of me, sitting on the floor in front of the fireplace stringing popcorn: I had forgotten about it until one day when I heard a song. The song, I had also forgotten. It emerged one evening from the shuffle function of a long playlist I had made several years ago. The song is called, *I Have Never Loved Someone*, performed by the band My Brightest Diamond, which is effectively the singer Shara Nova. The song appears to have been written to her son. I don't know if she has a son – on Wikipedia it says she has one child – but it doesn't matter. Son, daughter: anybody listening will hear a song from a mother to a child, and when I listen, I hear it through my heart for my own sons.

It is an absurdly simple song that ends with the mother promising that when she dies she will find a way, through the breeze, the warmth of the sun, the rain, any damn way, to send the child a message, an eternal message, an embracing message, surpassing time and space. And you think before she says the words that the message will be, *I love you*. Of course. What else? The simple song with the simple message of a million other songs. But *I love you* is not what she sings. She sings, *you're okay*.

You're okay.

And when I hear the words of this song that maybe is not as simple as it seems, I think *you're okay* might very well be the most precious gift a parent can offer a child. *I love you* is powerful. *You don't have to be anything but who you are to deserve love* is life-changing.

World-changing. Because it's not just parents who can give such a gift; any one of us can give it to anyone. Not everyone. But a lot of someones. And sometimes to ourselves. Who we are now and also who we used to be.

What is the more radical rerouting of the ruts in my brain: change or acceptance?

Here is a sentence that might be true: I have tended toward emotional sleeve-wearing for a long, long time and I could try to change it, but I could also try to come to terms with it. Acceptance, like compassion, does not appear to be a state you ever get to. It's like always you're on some point in the road toward getting there, working on it, some days further along than other days. Allowing for backtracking, for detours and a wrong turn or two. It takes practice. Lots of practice. A lifetime.

My mother was Miss Chattanooga in 1951. If you knew my mother you might be surprised, because she didn't seem like a beauty queen type. This is true. She never was the beauty queen type. She didn't actually set out to enter a beauty contest, never dreamed of winning, she did it as a favor to some college friends who were looking to sponsor a contestant. Then she won. She was just that beautiful and that talented. I imagine that to my mother at the time, the Miss Chattanooga beauty pageant was closer to a lark, less important than everything else that made up her busy young life, although it most certainly it was the sort of thing that would have pleased her own mother. Only later would it turn out to be the exact opposite of what a feminist would be proud of, and so by the time I was old enough to know that my mother had once been Miss Chattanooga, she was both embarrassed and irritated by some of the people she grew up with who continued -- for decades, really - to congratulate her on what she considered a trivial non-event.

When I turned 19, I was invited to the Cotton Ball, which would have required me to acquire both a long evening gown to walk around in and some male escort to walk around with me, in a kind of pageant to declare myself eligible in a stable of marriageable young women. I think my mother and I viewed the Cotton Ball in the context of her Miss Chattanooga story – how could we not? Both of us were certain to the core that women should not be objects for display. My worth absolutely never was going to be tied to any such measure as "marriageability," even symbolically. The mothers of several of my friends made them attend because it was the thing to do, to meet the expectations of polite, well-meaning society, but thankfully mine said, go or not go, it's your life. I did not go.

It was not difficult for me to see my mother as my role model.

When she was a girl, my mother remembers making a point of sitting next to black people on city buses because she did not want to be associated with the racists. She knew a lot of them, these racists. My mother had seen what Jim Crow was up to and knew it was wrong, and she did not want anybody mistaking her for some-body who did not know it was wrong. I asked her one time: how did she know? It wasn't like her family was particularly enlightened; certainly not the culture around her in Arkansas and Mississippi and Tennessee, where she spent some part of her childhood. She's never been able to answer that question. She just knew. All through the summer of 1973, she and I sat in front of the television and watched the Watergate hearings together. Together we were breath-less, waiting for justice.

One of us is still waiting.

My mother was a firecracker and a firebrand. Her moral compass never wavered. She was a sponge for information, for adventure, for beauty. She was a bright light, a beacon, for many people for a long time. I don't know how many people can say they are proud of their mothers, but I am one. I am and always have been proud to be the daughter of Charlotte Elaine Walker Landis.

And now she's worse. As always, it's hard to say exactly how, even as it's undeniable. For one thing, she's started to complain of being dizzy all the time. My dad, along with their doctor, is working on changing up medications, changing up dosages, plus he's watching over her hydration and diet, and some days it looks as if some of that might be helping. Other days, not so much. Could this Alzheimer's be creeping into dizzy-making brain regions? There's no way to know.

She's dizzy and she's weak and she's tired. More and more my mother goes entire days without getting dressed. She doesn't want to get dressed. She'll wear the same nightgown under the same bathrobe with the same socks and slippers for a week. She'll still work a crossword puzzle, still remembers lyrics to old songs, but mostly what she wants to do all day, every day, is take naps and watch re-runs of *Cheers*. So far, she has run through every episode of the entire series, twice. She does not remember she's watched any of them. She laughs, out loud, at the same jokes, over and over, as if she'd never heard them before. Almost every moment of her life she lives in the moment where she is. It's like the guy in *Memento*. It's like every day is Groundhog day.

Consider solitaire. My mother picks up the old, worn deck of cards that lives by her place at the kitchen table every time she sits down. Every time. For as long as I can remember, long before anybody ever thought of Alzheimer's, she was picking up those cards. (She'll change decks only after the cards begin to disintegrate.) Solitaire is what my mother does with her hands when she sits at the kitchen table, like a cigarette habit, like knitting, like scrolling on a phone. So on a recent visit to our house, when she didn't have her cards with her, Bruce asked if she would like some.

Why? She could not imagine why she would need a deck of cards.

In case you want to play solitaire.

Why would I want to play solitaire?

Because you play solitaire every day.

No I don't.

That's living in the moment.

If my father is not in the room with her, she'll have to ask a dozen times, where is he?

If her dog is not in the room with her, she'll have to ask a dozen times, where is she?

She cannot keep the answer in her head for more than a few seconds. And so my father stays disappeared, and the dog stays disappeared, until they return.

For her 90th birthday last December we threw two parties, one with friends and a second with our family. Already she's forgotten the parties. She forgot Christmas. She does not remember she is 90. She does not remember who the Beatles were. She does not ask for Aretha Franklin anymore. She is breaking my heart.

Need I tell you who the hero is?

My father understands what is required to keep my mother's mind from falling into itself. He has maintained the patience and humor to include her in the running of the house. Does she want to help with dinner? Does she want to wash the dishes? Occasionally he can coax her out to take a walk even when she doesn't want to, and he does not sound as bossy about it as I do. Her dignity is important to him. He does not tell her she can't have another cookie.

If anyone might need a tutorial on how to take care of a woman with Alzheimer's, I would point to my father.

He has become the keeper of the social calendar and of friendships. Two or three times a week, he arranges to meet friends for dinner. Even through the pandemic, he stayed connected to friends inside social bubbles, on porches and decks. When friends come over he will cook for them out of his new collection of cookbooks. Often my mother will not remember they are coming, and so he'll have to remind her to get dressed.

She will not want to get dressed. She will not want to have company, and sometimes she won't remember who the company is, and she might get mad at my dad for making her get off the couch. She'll get mad and pout, like a two-year-old gets mad, which can be charming and a little funny unless you're the one who has to deal with it every day.

But then – it's like a magic trick -- when friends walk in the door, my mother transforms. Suddenly she can keep up with conversations. Make jokes. Banter. Somehow my mother still loves a party, even these days when she appears increasingly confused.

I have no doubt that my mother's decline would have gone much, much faster if my father did not have the wisdom and patience and energy to fill her days, her life, with friends. She can play a little piano. She can work a crossword puzzle. Sometimes she cheats, but she still knows how to cheat. She still knows who we are.

That this disease is infinitely strange may make it interesting. But for me, it's heartbreaking.

(60+26)/2

Here I have come to the end of this little book. Now as I write this sentence, I am several years past 60 already and growing accustomed to living in my sixth decade; it's not such a shock to say my age these days. I'm starting to wonder if those youngsters in their 50s even know a damn thing. I will be okay in my 60s. I will want to make it to 70.

I did not know when I started this book if I would finish it. I did not keep track of how many times I stopped writing. Stopped because I was convinced such a book was ill-conceived from the get-go, one more failed project. So many times. I stopped writing and had to force myself to gear up again. Sit down, breathe, make myself write one sentence and then another, without the fuel of confidence to help. I have been reluctant to finish. Afraid to finish. Not sure I had it in me to finish.

One sentence and then another, and then the next one after that. I have been writing for a long, long time. So far, I have not found a way to quit, but through this book I may have accidentally written myself into a shift in my relationship to writing. Something has changed. It's a feeling of absence, the absence of so much struggle, so much desperation, so much wincing. I am open to the possibility that I do not have to play the game by its current rules. I am becoming aware that no one is preventing me from writing on my own terms and for my own goals. Because someday I will die. Which day, I don't know, but one day. How then is it not reasonable to ask, what am I doing this for? Who am I doing this for?

From that angle, I can see that writing does not have to be my career, nor does it have to dictate who I am. External feedback is nice, but is it critical?

I have never asked that question. Instead, I carried around a heavy load of unquestioned assumptions. What will happen if I sever writing from all that bullshit? When I defined writing as my career -- as my identity -- I gave myself a narrow ledge to stand on and tons of ways to fail.

So I finished. With a pinch of doggedness and smidgen of audacity, I wrote myself another book. Along the way, of course, I learned some math.

Math!

There would have been no book without the math. But then, I can't swear I would have learned the math without the book, because it took some prodding to sit down and work all those math problems. Working math problems gave me something to write about, and that, it turns out, became my carrot, my reward.

Now look at me. I am not innumerate anymore! Fractions don't scare me. Percentages can't humiliate me. Word problems are not out of my grasp. It feels like I'm one of those normal people who took math in school and retained, not all of it, but enough to get by.

I have re-set. Two trains are leaving the station, you say? Hand me a pencil and a piece of paper.

For a brain exercise, I recommend it. Yes, ma'am. Math will put your brain through some things. Sharpen your focus. Shake up your thinking. In between those word games, the Spanish lessons, the piano lessons, the weight classes, and the working of the crossword puzzles, try solving for X and see how you feel.

Will it prevent Alzheimer's disease?

I don't know. Nobody knows.

At least I have done what I set out to do, and along the way I managed to answer most of my questions about math and why it was always so hard for me.

I believe I was born with a brain that does not think mathematically.

I am not particularly interested in puzzles.

I think math is different from other subjects because it is unforgiving.

I think math is the same as other subjects because moving to more complex levels depends on mastering basics. Same with English or Spanish or tennis or basketball.

Forgetting trigonometry is not somehow worse than forgetting what John Locke said.

I don't believe being good at math has anything to do with gender.

I believe I did not always have the best math teachers.

I believe my teachers did not have the all the tools they might have needed to teach math to students like me.

I believe I was afraid of my teachers.

I believe if I'd had better teachers I might have been better at math.

Better, but not great. Because I wasn't born with that kind of brain. *(See above.)*

I may have a mild case of synesthesia. I don't believe that's why math is hard for me.

I believe I can get better at math than I currently am.

I believe I could have learned more math than I did.

And I believe that's on me.

I believe there is a limit to how far I can go in math.

I believe fear held me back.

I don't believe this is a book about math.

References

How To Become A Superager, by Lisa Feldman Barrett, New York Times, December 2016

Fractions: Where it All Goes Wrong, Robert S. Siegler, November 28, 2017 Scientific American

THE GROWTH MINDSET, Dr. Carol Dweck

DEMENTIAL REIMAGINED, Dr. Tia Powell

Alzheimer's Association

IN PURSUIT OF MEMORY, Joseph Jebelli

Math With Bad Drawings, Ben Orlin

Dan Finkle, MATH FOR LOVE

Are Boys Better than Girls at Math, Colleen Ganley, Scientific American, August 14, 2018

Math + Culture = Gender Gap, Beth Azor, July 2010 American Psychology Association

HALF EMPTY, David Rakoff

ESSAYS AFTER 80, Donald Hall

I Have Never Loved Someone, My Brightest Diamond

Acknowledgements

Never could I have written this book without the expertise and encouragement of friends, readers, and math teachers. They were my guides into math world, my cheerleaders who believed when I did not. Thank you to Mary Smith, Grier Novinger, Carl Wagner, Alice Ingle, Lucy Tyler, Sharon Rasch, Brenda Rasch, Julie Wolf, Kerry Madden, Christy Mabe Scott, Charles Landis, Emily Landis, Sheila Wood Navaro, Sylvia Walker, Flossie McNabb, and Judy Tipton.

A special thank you to Claire Roberts for her tireless work and support.

I remain inspired and enriched by my family: my sons, my daughters-in-law, my grandsons, my brother and his family. I am especially indebted to my father, Charlie Landis, and of course my mother, Charlotte. I have been, and always will be, amazed and grateful for the love and support of my husband, Bruce. Without him, this little book would have remained in the bowels of my laptop.

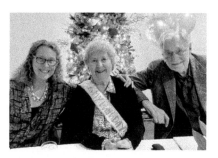

The author with her parents on
the occasion of her mother's
90th birthday

Catherine is the author of two published novels, SOME DAYS THERE'S PIE (St. Martin's Press, 2001) and HARVEST (Thomas Dunne Books, 2004). She is the mother of two grown sons and the grandmother of two grandsons. She is a runner, hiker, activist for progressive causes, and a pretty good cook. She lives in Knoxville Tennessee with her husband.

Lightning Source UK Ltd.
Milton Keynes UK
UKHW020757180422
401668UK00009B/707